Neurology in Practice

T0136765

Neurology in Practice

Fifth Edition

Y. L. Yu 余毓靈
MD (HK), FRCP, FRCPE, FRACP, FHKCP, FHKAM (Medicine)

J. K. Y. Fong 方嘉揚
MBBS (HK), FRCP, FRCPE, FHKCP, FHKAM (Medicine)

S. L. Ho 何樹良
MD (Wales), FRCP, FRCPE, FRCPG, FHKCP, FHKAM (Medicine)

R. T. F. Cheung 張德輝
MBBS (HK), PhD (W Ont), FRCP, FRCPE, FRCPG, FHKCP, FHKAM (Medicine)

K. H. Chan 陳灌豪
MD (HK), PhD (HK), FRCPG, FHKCP, FHKAM (Medicine)

HKU
PRESS
香港大學出版社

Hong Kong University Press
The University of Hong Kong
Pokfulam Road
Hong Kong
www.hkupress.org

ISBN 978-988-8390-73-1 (*Paperback*)

British Library Cataloguing-in-Publication Data
A catalogue record for this book is available from the British Library.

10 9 8 7 6 5 4 3 2 1

Printed and bound by Paramount Printing Co., Ltd. in Hong Kong, China

Contents

Foreword to the Second Edition

In the preface to the first edition of this textbook, Dr Y. L. Yu mentioned that most medical students, and indeed trainees, consider neurology a difficult subject. This is partly due to the intricacies of neuroanatomy and also because, apart from a few disorders such as the cerebrovascular diseases, patients with neurological problems are not that commonly seen in a general medical ward. Furthermore, sections on neurology in standard textbooks are either too brief or too all-encompassing for the medical student. This textbook is neither. The chapters are clearly written and presented, and there are many helpful tables and diagrams. The information is also very up-to-date.

This book covers the majority of common neurological disorders, in particular those seen in this area of the world. It emphasizes aetiology, clinical features and approach to diagnosis, and outlines management.

The chapter on the cranial nerves with examples of their common disorders is logical and useful. The authors' personal views and practical advice based on experience are a valuable aspect of this textbook. For example, it is emphasized that only a small proportion of patients with headache need investigations. The chapter on infections is appropriately more detailed, useful for this area of the world and important in view of the increasing number of patients with compromised immunity. Topical and newer entities, such as Alzheimer's disease, prion, and mitochondrial disorders, are also discussed.

This textbook assumes basic knowledge of neuroanatomy, and certain details of more sophisticated investigations and treatment must be sought elsewhere. Accordingly, at the end of the book there are recommendations for further reading. This is an eminently

readable and succinct modern short textbook of neurology, cov-
ering the common and important topics interspersed with sound,
practical advice and guidelines to diagnosis and management. It can
be highly recommended to both undergraduate and postgraduate
students and medical practitioners, and the authors deserve our
compliments and thanks.

Professor Sir David Todd
Hong Kong
June 1997

Preface to the Fifth Edition

This book was first published in 1994. In the past two decades, there have been transformative advances in clinical neurology. Neurogenetics has shed light on many hitherto mysterious disorders. Sophisticated neuroimaging has enabled precise anatomical localization of lesions and elucidation of physiology and pathology. Cerebrovascular disease is now eminently treatable, with thrombolysis and endovascular procedures taking the lead. Effective treatments are available for movement disorders, demyelinating disease, and autoimmune encephalitis. With neurorehabilitation, patients with stroke and trauma of the nervous system can enjoy better quality of life.

Amid these advances, clinical practice remains central. Thus, enhancement of the practice of neurology continues to be the aim of this book. We emphasize proper clinical methodology and application of evidence-based knowledge for effective management. Two new chapters have been added; they are Chapter 5 'Disorders of Cerebrospinal Fluid Dynamics' and Chapter 10 'Autoimmune Disorders of the Nervous System'. All existing chapters have been updated with knowledge gained from major advances in neuroscience.

Over the years, readership has extended from medical students to trainees in internal medicine and neurology, physicians, nurses, and allied health workers. We are indebted to them for sharing their feedback with us in the course of preparing this and previous editions.

Y. L. Yu, J. K. Y. Fong
S. L. Ho, R. T. F. Cheung, K. H. Chan
Hong Kong
March 2017

Preface to the First Edition

This handbook was conceived because of popular demand and is the collaborative effort of members of the Department of Medicine, the University of Hong Kong.

Whilst there are plenty of good neurology textbooks on the market, students often find neurology a subject hard to master and neurological diagnosis difficult to make. There are perhaps a number of reasons. Textbooks do not usually adopt a practical approach as required in clinical practice, and the emphasis on certain diseases applies more to Caucasian than Chinese patients. More importantly, students do not seem to appreciate that neurology, more so than other disciplines, is best learnt by applying book knowledge in clinical situations.

Thus, the objective of this handbook is to enhance the practice of neurology. To this end, common neurological disorders have been selected, and the focus is on key concepts, local disease patterns and characteristics, as well as accurate diagnosis and effective management. Moreover, for important topics, recent advances are included. The references section provides a source of in-depth information for interested readers. Thus, this handbook aims at medical education in the broader sense rather than rote learning of facts. It must also be emphasized that it is intended to complement rather than replace standard textbooks.

It is hoped that this handbook will not only promote students' interest in the intellectual challenge presented by neurology, but will also stimulate the enquiring mind to prepare for a lifetime of continuous medical education.

There is certainly room for improvement in this first edition, and comments and suggestions from colleagues and students are welcome. The authors and editor are grateful to Miss Miranda Ho, who has provided meticulous and skilful secretarial assistance in the preparation of the manuscripts.

Y. L. Yu
Hong Kong
June 1994

Abbreviations

ABG	arterial blood gases
Ach	acetylcholine
AChR	acetylcholine receptor
anti-AChR	anti-acetylcholine receptor antibodies
AD, AR	autosomal dominant, autosomal recessive
ADEM	acute disseminated encephalomyelitis
ADL	activities of daily living
ADP, ATP	adenosine diphosphate, adenosine triphosphate
AED(s)	antiepileptic drug(s)
AF	atrial fibrillation
AFB	acid-fast bacilli
AIDP	acute inflammatory demyelinating polyradiculoneuropathy
AIDS	acquired immunodeficiency syndrome
ALS	amyotrophic lateral sclerosis
APTT	activated partial thromboplastin time
ATT	anti-tetanus toxoid
AVM	arteriovenous malformation
BAEP	brainstem auditory evoked potentials
BBB	blood-brain-barrier
BMT	bone marrow transplantation
BP	blood pressure
BSE	bovine spongiform encephalopathy
CBC	complete blood count
CIDP	chronic inflammatory demyelinating polyradiculoneuropathy
CJD	Creutzfeldt-Jakob disease
vCJD	variant Creutzfeldt-Jakob disease

CK(-MB)	creatine kinase (-myocardial band)
CMV	cytomegalovirus
CNS	central nervous system
COMT	catechol-O-methyltransferase
CPS	complex partial seizures
CSF	cerebrospinal fluid
CSM/R	cervical spondylotic myelopathy/ radiculopathy
CT	computed tomography
CTS	carpal tunnel syndrome
CVD	cerebrovascular disease
CXR	chest radiography
DIC	disseminated intravascular coagulopathy
DM	diabetes mellitus
DMD	Duchenne muscular dystrophy
DVT	deep vein thrombosis
EBV	Epstein-Barr virus
ECG	electrocardiogram
EC-IC	extracranial-intracranial
EDSS	Expanded Disability Status Scale
EEG	electroencephalography
ELISA	enzyme-linked immunosorbent assay
EMG	electromyography
ENT	ear, nose, and throat
EP	evoked potentials
ESR	erythrocyte sedimentation rate
FTA-Abs	fluorescent treponemal antibody-absorbed test
FVC	forced vital capacity
GBS	Guillain-Barré syndrome
GCS	Glasgow Coma Scale
GI	gastrointestinal
GPI	general paralysis of the insane
HBV	hepatitis-B virus
HIV	human immunodeficiency virus
HLA	human leucocyte antigens
HMSN	hereditary motor sensory neuropathy
HSAN	hereditary sensory autonomic neuropathy

HSV	herpes simplex virus
5-HT	5-hydroxytryptamine (serotonin)
HTLV	human T-lymphotrophic virus
ICA	internal carotid artery
ICH	intracerebral haemorrhage
ICP	intracranial pressure
ICU	intensive care unit
IgA/G/M	immunoglobulin A/G/M
IM(I)	intramuscular (injection)
INR	international normalized ratio
ISS	ischaemic stroke
IV(I)	intravenous (injection)
IVIG	intravenous immunoglobulins
JC virus	John Cunningham virus
KF	Kayser-Fleischer
KSS	Kearne-Sayre syndrome
LFT	liver function tests
LGI-1	Leucine-rich glioma inactivated-1
LMN/UMN	lower/upper motor neurone
LMWH	low-molecular-weight heparin
LOC	loss of consciousness
LP	lumbar puncture
MAP	muscle action potentials
cMAP	compound muscle action potentials
MELAS	mitochondrial encephalomyopathy, lactic acidosis, and stroke-like episodes
MERRF	myoclonus epilepsy with ragged red fibres
MG	myasthenia gravis
MMSE	Mini-Mental State Examination
MND	motor neurone disease
MRC	Medical Research Council
MRI/A/S	magnetic resonance imaging/angiography spectroscopy
MS	multiple sclerosis
MSA	multisystem atrophy
MuSK	muscle-specific kinase
anti-MuSK	anti-muscle specific kinase antibodies

NCS/V	nerve conduction study/velocity
NMDA	N-methyl-D-aspartic acid
NMDAR	N-methyl-D-aspartate receptor
anti-NMDAR	anti-N-methyl-D-aspartate receptor antibodies
NMJ	neuromuscular junction
NMOSD	neuromyelitis optica spectrum disorders
NPC	nasopharyngeal carcinoma
NSAID(s)	non-steroidal anti-inflammatory drug(s)
OA	osteoarthritis
OB	oligoclonal bands
OSA	obstructive sleep apnoea
PAN	polyarteritis nodosa
PCR	polymerase chain reaction
PET	positron emission tomography
PML	progressive multifocal leucoencephalopathy
PNS	peripheral nervous system
PPMS	primary progressive multiple sclerosis
PRMS	progressive relapsing multiple sclerosis
PT	prothrombin time
PTA	post-traumatic amnesia
REM	rapid eye movements
RFT	renal function tests
RNS	repetitive nerve stimulation
RRMS	relapsing-remitting multiple sclerosis
SAH	subarachnoid haemorrhage
SAP	sensory action potentials
SC(I)	subcutaneous (injection)
SEP	somatosensory evoked potentials
SIADH	syndrome of inappropriate anti-diuretic hormone
SLE	systemic lupus erythematosus
SMA	spinal muscular atrophy
SPECT	single photon emission computed tomography
SPMS	secondary progressive multiple sclerosis
SSPE	subacute sclerosing panencephalitis

SUDEP	sudden unexpected death in epilepsy
TB	tuberculosis/tuberculous
TBM	tuberculous meningitis
TIA	transient ischaemic attack(s)
tPA	tissue plasminogen activator
TPHA	treponemal haemagglutination test
TSH	thyroid stimulating hormone
VDRL	Venereal Disease Research Laboratory test
VEP	visual evoked potentials
VNS	vagus nerve stimulation
VZV	varicella zoster virus
WBC	white blood cells
XL	X-linked
XR	X-ray

About the Authors

Y. L. Yu is a neurologist in private practice and is Honorary Clinical Professor at the University of Hong Kong and Honorary Consultant at Hong Kong Sanatorium & Hospital. His previous appointments include Registrar and Senior Registrar at National Hospital for Neurology and Neurosurgery, Queen Square, London, and Reader in Neurology, Department of Medicine, University of Hong Kong.

J. K. Y. Fong is a neurologist in private practice and is Consultant Neurologist at Hong Kong Adventist Hospital. His past appointments include Honorary Clinical Assistant Professor at the University of Hong Kong and Honorary Consultant (Neurology) in the Department of Medicine at Ruttonjee Hospital, Senior Medical Officer at Queen Mary Hospital, and Honorary Research Fellow at UCL Institute of Neurology, Queen Square, London.

S. L. Ho is the Henry G. Leong Professor in Neurology and Division Chief (Neurology) at the University of Hong Kong. He is also Honorary Consultant at Queen Mary Hospital and Tung Wah Hospital. A graduate of the University of Wales College of Medicine, he received his general medical training in Coventry and Manchester, and subsequently training in neurology in Birmingham, England. He was Registrar and Clinical Research Fellow at the Department of Neurology, University of Birmingham.

R. T. F. Cheung is the Lee Man-Chiu Professor in Neuroscience at the University of Hong Kong, Director of Acute Stroke Services at Hong Kong West Cluster, and Honorary Consultant at Queen Mary Hospital and Tung Wah Hospital. His previous appointments include Clinical Fellow in Neurology at the Department of Clinical Neurological Sciences, University of Western Ontario, and Staff Neurologist of the North American Symptomatic Carotid Endarterectomy Trial, Robarts Research Institute, Ontario.

K. H. Chan is Clinical Associate Professor in the Department of Medicine at the University of Hong Kong and Honorary Consultant at Queen Mary Hospital. His previous appointments include Research Fellow in Autoimmune Neurology at the Mayo Clinic, Mayo Medical School, Minnesota, and Clinical Assistant Professor at the University of Hong Kong.

1 Approach to Neurological Diagnosis

Neurology is the branch of medical science which deals with the nervous system in both its normal and diseased states. Clinical neurology is the application of the basic neurosciences, in particular neuroanatomy, neurophysiology, and neurochemistry in patient management.

Most students and practitioners tend to shy away from neurology allegedly because it is perceived to be difficult. In fact, solving a neurological problem can be the most fascinating exercise in detection and logical deduction in clinical medicine. This demands an organized line of thought, a clear plan to be followed, and a specific aim at each stage of the investigation. As long as a proper approach is adopted, neurological diagnosis can be a straightforward and rewarding exercise.

When one approaches a patient with a neurological problem, three vital questions ought to be asked:
1. Where is/are the lesion(s)?
2. What is/are the probable underlying pathological condition(s)?
3. Is the disorder neurological or functional?

History

History taking is not a haphazard activity; it should focus on the three questions. With care, the diagnosis can be made from the history alone in many cases. In others, the history will direct one to focus on certain aspects of neurological examination. This is important, since the patient may not be able to cooperate if one pursues every fine detail of a full neurological examination. In certain diseases, such as epilepsy and headache, the history is crucial for the diagnosis because physical examination and investigation are often negative.

Relatives or eyewitnesses should be interviewed as far as possible since many patients may not be aware of the incident and symptoms, or are unable to give a full history because of impaired cognition and/or dysphasia.

The history can be unnecessarily lengthy if there is no emphasis, but details should be obtained in relevant areas. The following items should be covered:

- Details of the presenting symptom
- Mode of onset: acute, subacute, insidious
- Duration
- Course of illness: static, intermittent, progressive
- Associated symptoms: positive and negative
- Possible causes or risk factors of the disease
- Psychological aspects
- Functional status: how well the patient copes with the disability
- Family history
- Social (including occupational) history

Physical examination

After history taking, one should have a good idea as to which functional aspects of the nervous system are affected, and detailed examination must be directed to the relevant areas. The examination will serve to confirm the diagnosis suggested by the history.

It cannot be over-emphasized that one must be systematic in the neurological examination; otherwise one will get lost or overlook some important tests. A proposed scheme is as follows.

General examination

This includes recognition of abnormal facies and peripheral signs. It may provide clues to the cause, risk factors or associated conditions of the neurological disorder. Examples are:

- Clubbing and lymphadenopathy in cerebral metastasis
- Blood pressure and heart rhythm in syncope
- Goitre and thyroid signs in myopathy and neuropathy
- Skin rash in dermatomyositis
- Nail fold changes in vasculitis

Non-neurological causes of 'neurological' symptoms and important co-morbid conditions may also be identified. Examples are:
- Ear and hearing abnormality in patients with dizziness
- Osteoarthritis of the hip in patients with leg weakness

Neurological examination

Neurological examination begins with observing the patient during history taking. Such observation provides information on higher mental functions. Patient's own interpretation of symptoms may reveal anxiety, depression, neurosis or delusion.

Components of a practical neurological examination:
- Higher mental functions (relatives' observations can be very helpful)
  - Assess impaired consciousness using Glasgow Coma Scale (see Table 12.2)
  - Orientation: place, time, person
  - Memory: – immediate recall
    - short-term
    - long-term
  - Serial 7: 100-7→93→86→79→72→65
  - Current knowledge
  - Mood
  - Insight
  - Speech – Language: ascertain handedness first, then content of speech; dysphasia may be expressive, receptive or global
    - Articulation: dysarthria
  - The Mini-Mental State Examination (MMSE) incorporates many of the above items and is widely used for screening cognitive deficits (see Table 11.2).
- Cranial nerves (see also Chapter 3)
  - I: any change in smell, test each side with aromatic, non-irritant materials
  - II: visual acuity, direct and indirect light reflexes, visual field, fundi
  - III, IV, VI: eye movements in different directions; check for diplopia, nystagmus, and gaze palsy

- V: facial sensation to pinprick and light touch in all three divisions of the trigeminal nerve, corneal reflex, power of jaw opening and closure, jaw jerk
- VII: facial symmetry, UMN and LMN facial weakness
- VIII: hearing acuity, Weber's and Rinne's test (256 Hz tuning fork)
- IX, X: any hoarseness of voice, symmetry of palatal movements, gag reflex
- XI: power of sternomastoid and trapezius
- XII: any deviation, wasting or fasciculation of tongue
- Motor examination of upper and lower limbs
  - Muscle bulk, tone, power (Tables 1.1 and 1.2), tendon reflexes, plantar response, coordination, gait
  - Differentiate between UMN and LMN signs
  - Segmental levels for reflexes: biceps (C5–6), supinator (C5–6), triceps (C7–8), finger jerks (C8–T1), knee (L3–4), ankle (S1–2)
- Sensations of upper and lower limbs
  - Pain, temperature, vibration (128 Hz tuning fork), joint position
  - Recognize pattern of sensory loss: peripheral nerve *vs* dermatome (Figure 1.1)
  - C5–T1 dermatomes over the upper limb: shoulder (C5), thumb (C6), middle finger (C7), little finger (C8), inner-upper arm (T1)
  - C4 and T2 are contiguous over sternal angle
  - Over the trunk: nipple (T4), xiphisternum (T7), umbilicus (T10), symphysis pubis (L1)
  - L2–S2 over the lower limb: upper outer thigh (L2), lower inner thigh (L3), inner lower leg (L4), anterior lower leg and foot (L5), lateral lower leg (S1), mid-strip of leg posteriorly (S2)
  - S3 over saddle region
  - S4–5 over perianal region

Table 1.1 Segmental innervation of upper limb muscles

Region	Muscle	C4	C5	C6	C7	C8	T1
Shoulder	Supraspinatus	✓	✓				
	Teres minor	✓	✓				
	Deltoid	✓	✓	✓			
	Infraspinatus	✓	✓	✓			
	Subscapularis		✓	✓			
	Teres major		✓	✓	✓		
Arm	Biceps		✓	✓			
	Brachialis		✓	✓			
	Coracobrachialis		✓	✓	✓		
	Triceps			✓	✓	✓	
	Anconeus				✓	✓	
Forearm	Supinator longus		✓	✓			
	Supinator brevis		✓	✓			
	Extensor carpi radialis			✓	✓		
	Pronator teres			✓	✓		
	Flexor carpi radialis			✓	✓		
	Flexor pollicis longus			✓	✓	✓	
	Abductor pollicis longus			✓	✓	✓	
	Extensor pollicis brevis				✓	✓	✓
	Extensor pollicis longus			✓	✓	✓	
	Extensor digitorum communis			✓	✓	✓	
	Extensor indicis			✓	✓	✓	
	Extensor carpi ulnaris			✓	✓	✓	
	Extensor digiti minimi			✓	✓	✓	
	Flexor digitorum superficialis				✓	✓	✓
	Flexor digitorum profundus				✓	✓	✓
	Pronator quadratus				✓	✓	✓
	Flexor carpi ulnaris				✓	✓	✓
	Palmaris longus				✓	✓	✓
Hand	Abductor pollicis brevis				✓	✓	✓
	Flexor pollicis brevis				✓	✓	✓
	Opponens pollicis				✓	✓	
	Flexor digiti minimi				✓	✓	✓
	Opponens digiti minimi				✓	✓	✓
	Adductor pollicis					✓	✓
	Palmaris brevis					✓	✓
	Abductor digiti minimi					✓	✓
	Lumbricals					✓	✓
	Interossei					✓	✓

Table 1.2 Segmental innervation of lower limb muscles

Region	Muscle	L1	L2	L3	L4	L5	S1	S2	S3
Hip	Iliopsoas	✓	✓	✓	✓	✓			
	Tensor fascia latae				✓	✓			
	Gluteus medius				✓	✓	✓		
	Gluteus minimus				✓	✓	✓		
	Quadratus femoris				✓	✓	✓		
	Gluteus maximus				✓	✓	✓		
	Obturator internus					✓	✓		
	Piriformis					✓	✓		
Thigh	Sartorius		✓	✓					
	Pectineus		✓	✓					
	Adductor longus		✓	✓					
	Quadriceps		✓	✓	✓				
	Gracilis		✓	✓	✓				
	Adductor brevis		✓	✓	✓				
	Obturator externus			✓	✓				
	Adductor magnus			✓	✓				
	Adductor minimus			✓	✓				
	Articularis genus			✓	✓				
	Semitendinosus				✓	✓	✓		
	Semimembranosus				✓	✓	✓		
	Biceps femoris				✓	✓	✓	✓	
Leg	Tibialis anterior				✓	✓			
	Extensor hallucis longus				✓	✓	✓		
	Popliteus				✓	✓	✓		
	Plantaris				✓	✓	✓		
	Extensor digitorum longus				✓	✓	✓		
	Soleus				✓	✓	✓	✓	
	Gastrocnemius				✓	✓	✓	✓	
	Peroneus longus					✓	✓		
	Peroneus brevis					✓	✓		
	Tibialis posterior					✓	✓	✓	
	Flexor digitorum longus					✓	✓	✓	✓
	Flexor hallucis longus					✓	✓	✓	✓
	Extensor hallucis brevis				✓	✓	✓		
Foot	Extensor digitorum brevis				✓	✓	✓		
	Flexor digitorum brevis					✓	✓		
	Abductor hallucis					✓	✓		
	Flexor hallucis brevis					✓	✓	✓	✓
	Lumbricals					✓	✓	✓	✓
	Abductor digiti minimi						✓	✓	✓
	Flexor digiti minimi brevis						✓	✓	✓
	Opponens digiti minimi						✓	✓	✓
	Quadratus plantae						✓	✓	✓
	Interossei						✓	✓	✓

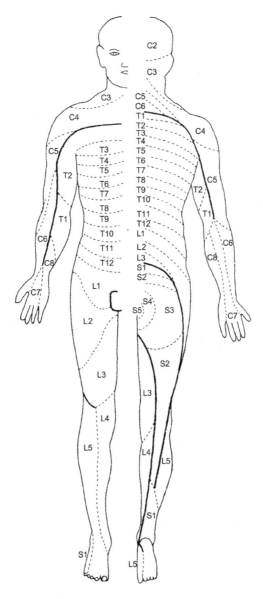

Figure 1.1 Dermatomes of the body, upper, and lower limbs.

Cardiovascular system

- Pulse
- Blood pressure
- Heart sounds and murmurs
- Arterial bruit

Respiratory system

Abdomen

Diagnosis

Upon completion of the examination, it should be possible to arrive at the diagnosis in most cases. There are two stages in the diagnosis: anatomical and pathological.

Anatomical diagnosis

The lesion(s) may be:
- Single, e.g., tumour in the brainstem
- Two or more but discrete, e.g., optic nerve and spinal cord lesions as in multiple sclerosis
- Diffuse, e.g., neurodegenerative disease or viral encephalomyelitis

Anatomical localization applies to single or multiple discrete lesions. The sites of the central (brain and spinal cord) and peripheral nervous systems are:

- Brain
  - Cerebral hemispheres
    - dominant
    - non-dominant } Anterior and middle cranial fossae
  - Brainstem
    - midbrain
    - pons
    - medulla oblongata
  - Cerebellum } Posterior cranial fossa
- Spinal cord
- Spinal root

- Plexus – brachial, lumbosacral
- Peripheral nerve
- Neuromuscular junction
- Muscle

The clinical features and relevant investigations for localization are tabulated (Tables 1.3–1.10). See also Chapter 18 for features of cortical dysfunction.

Table 1.3   Hemisphere lesion

Clinical features
Impaired mentation, dysphasia (dominant), dyspraxia (non-dominant)
Homonymous visual field defects
Contralateral UMN facial weakness, dysarthria
Contralateral UMN limb weakness
Contralateral sensory disturbance
Conjugate gaze deviation towards lesion
Focal seizures

Investigations
MRI or CT brain, EEG

A UMN lesion refers to a lesion either at the cortex or corticobulbar/corticospinal tract. This may give rise to contralateral facial weakness with relative sparing of the upper facial muscles which are innervated bilaterally. The UMN lesion may also give rise to contralateral limb weakness with spasticity and exaggerated tendon reflexes.

Table 1.4   Posterior fossa lesion

Clinical features
Cranial nerve deficits
Bilateral or unilateral UMN limb weakness
Bilateral or unilateral sensory disturbance
Cerebellar ataxia, nystagmus
Conjugate gaze deviation away from lesion

Investigations
MRI or CT brain, BAEP

NB: Signs of raised intracranial pressure tend to appear early for mass lesions in the posterior fossa.

Table 1.5   Spinal cord lesion

Clinical features
UMN limb weakness below lesion – unilateral or bilateral
LMN limb weakness at level of lesion – unilateral or bilateral
Pattern of sensory deficits – level, glove and stocking, suspended,
    dissociated
Sphincter disturbance

Investigations
MRI spine*, XR spine, SEP, CSF analysis

*If MRI not available, myelogram or CT myelogram is an alternative.

A LMN lesion refers to a lesion of the motor neurone or its axons. Depending on the site (brainstem or spinal cord), it may give rise to ipsilateral facial weakness affecting the upper and lower facial muscles or ipsilateral limb weakness with hypotonia and reduced or absent tendon reflexes.

Table 1.6   Spinal root lesion

Clinical features
Segmental LMN weakness and sensory deficits
Autonomic disturbance

Investigations
NCS, EMG, SEP, XR spine, MRI spine*, CSF analysis

*If MRI not available, myelogram or CT myelogram is an alternative.

Table 1.7   Plexus lesion

Clinical features
Multi-segmental LMN weakness and sensory deficits
Autonomic disturbance

Investigations
NCS, EMG, SEP, MRI, CSF analysis

Table 1.8   Peripheral nerve lesion

Clinical features	
LMN weakness	Patterns – symmetrical sensorimotor
Sensory deficits	mononeuritis multiplex
Autonomic disturbance	mononeuropathy

Investigations
NCS, EMG, CSF analysis, nerve biopsy

Table 1.9   Neuromuscular junction lesion

Clinical features
Weakness without wasting – generalized or focal
Fatiguability or post-exertion reinforcement
Autonomic disturbance

Investigations
Tensilon test, Anti-AChR, CK, thyroid function, repetitive stimulation

Table 1.10   Myopathy

Clinical features
Weakness, wasting or pseudohypertrophy, generalized or in groups
Muscle pain
Tendon reflexes may be normal or reduced

Investigations
CK, immune markers, muscle biopsy

Pathological diagnosis

Having made the anatomical diagnosis, the pathological diagnosis has to be postulated. The clues are the mode of onset, duration, and progression of symptoms. For example, a vascular lesion is usually of sudden onset and reaches the maximum intensity within a short time. A tumour is usually of insidious onset and progressive deterioration. Other clues are also helpful. For example, a familial history would indicate a hereditary aetiology. A pre-existing collagen disease would suggest an autoimmune basis of the lesion. It is often helpful to go through the list of likely pathology:

- Congenital
- Hereditary

- Inflammatory: infective, granulomatous, autoimmune
- Demyelinating
- Vascular
- Degenerative
- Neoplastic: benign, malignant
- Traumatic
- Idiopathic

Investigations

After a clinical diagnosis has been arrived at, the next steps are to confirm it and to obtain more information in order to plan the management. Investigations (Tables 1.3–1.10) are organized with these aims in mind. To be cost-effective, they should be specific and relevant. Such targeting can only be achieved with a sound clinical diagnosis.

Common neurological symptoms and their differential diagnosis

Headache (see Chapter 4)

Facial pain (see Chapter 3)

Dizziness

This is a common symptom which may be due to systemic or vestibular disturbance. Distinction has to be made from loss or lapse of consciousness. Associated symptoms of vertigo and disequilibrium, if present, should be elicited.

Systemic disturbance
    presyncope
    hyperventilation
    anaemia
    cardiac arrhythmia
    drug-induced, e.g., bromocriptine, levodopa, methyldopa
    electrolyte disturbance, e.g., hyponatraemia

Vestibular disturbance
   Peripheral
   labyrinthitis
   Meniere's disease

   Central
   brainstem/cerebellar lesion
   vertebrobasilar stroke
   cerebello-pontine angle tumours
   demyelination

Altered consciousness

This state includes complete and partial, prolonged and brief disturbance of consciousness. Details of relevant features during the episode should be obtained from the patient or relatives. Many causes of impaired consciousness apply (see Chapter 12).
   epileptic seizures, generalized or complex partial
   stroke
   cardiogenic syncope
   metabolic/endocrine, especially hypoglycaemia
   intoxication/drug overdose, e.g., alcohol, substance abuse
   neoplastic
   functional disorders

Visual impairment (see Chapter 3)

Ptosis

Unilateral
   III nerve palsy
   Horner's syndrome
   MG

Bilateral
   MG
   myopathy

Diplopia (see Chapter 3)

Deafness (see Chapter 3)

Dysphagia

Structural lesion (symptoms worse with solid food)
    oesophageal carcinoma or stricture

Impaired neural control (symptoms worse with fluid)
    bulbar palsy (see Chapter 3)
    pseudobulbar palsy, e.g., stroke, MND
    neuromuscular junction, e.g., MG, botulism
    neuropathy, e.g., AIDP

Tremors (see Chapter 8)

Gait disturbance in the absence of limb weakness

Apraxic:	diffuse cerebral disease
	subcortical ischaemia or demyelination
	normal pressure hydrocephalus
Ataxic:	cerebellar lesion especially midline
	loss of joint position sense, e.g., neurosyphilis, sub-acute combined degeneration of cord, diabetic neuropathy
Shuffling:	parkinsonism

Sensory disturbance in extremities

peripheral neuropathy
cervical myelopathy
functional disorders

Simulated neurological manifestations

It is not uncommon for patients with psychogenic disorders to present with various neurological (and/or other somatic) symptoms.

Common simulated neurological features include impaired cognition, amnesia, seizures, blindness, diplopia, aphonia, limb weakness, gait disturbance, tics, tremor, dystonia, pain, and paraesthesia. In these cases, a neurological explanation of the symptoms and signs cannot be found even after thorough examination and investigation. The patient may derive some primary gain from expressing the suppressed unconscious conflict. Avoidance of unpleasant situations, compensation issues, and undue attention from family and carers may constitute secondary gain. A comprehensive psychosocial history from friends and family is essential.

The diagnosis of psychogenic illnesses should only be made after all reasonable steps have been undertaken to exclude organic disorders. Misdiagnosing an organic condition for a psychogenic illness may have serious consequences such as negligence claims (see Chapter 20). Repeated visits may be required before the diagnosis can be made. Do not rush into invasive diagnostic tests or potentially harmful therapeutic interventions as these may bring about more complicated problems. A trial of physiotherapy, psychotherapy, anxiolytic, or antidepressant may be helpful. Consider referral to psychologists or psychiatrists.

The following clues suggest the manifestations are psychogenic in nature:

- The pattern of deficits does not conform to neuroanatomy or neurophysiology.
- Multiple somatic complaints
- Findings on formal examination are inconsistent with functional observation, which is especially useful when the patient is unaware of being observed.
- Variable findings in different examinations

Psychogenic limb weakness
  - No muscle wasting or atrophy
  - Normal reflexes and tone
  - Give-way weakness or fluctuating weakness
  - Extensor and flexor muscles equally weak
  - Simultaneous contraction of the agonist and antagonist muscles when executing a movement

Psychogenic movement disorders
  - Abrupt onset, atypical pattern, paroxysmal symptoms
  - Inconsistency over time
  - Entrainment of tremor to the examiner's suggested rate
  - Spontaneous remissions
  - Disappearance when distracted
  - Aggravation during formal examination
  - Response to placebo, psychotherapy or suggestion

Psychogenic seizure (see Chapter 7)

Always bear in mind the following:
- Organic and psychogenic disorders may coexist.
- Delirium and dementia are due to organic disorders.
- Cerebrovascular disease, brain tumour, epilepsy, Parkinson's disease, Alzheimer's disease, multiple sclerosis, and Huntington's disease can produce anxiety and depression.
- Substance misuse (e.g., alcohol, recreational drugs) can lead to psychogenic and neurological complications.
- Psychosomatic disorders consist of hysteria, somatization disorders, somatoform pain disorders, and neurasthenia. They commonly present with fatigue, dizziness, headache or pain attributed to physical illness.
- A patient with factitious disorder repeatedly induces the symptoms or signs of disease in the absence of any psychiatric or physical disorder.

2 Neurodiagnostic Tests

Neuroimaging

Computed tomography (CT)

CT measures attenuation of radiation for small volume elements (voxels) and uses computer to generate a 2-D picture composed of a matrix of voxels. High-density structures (e.g., bone) are white and low-density tissues (e.g., air, fat) are dark or black.

Advanced spiral scanner and multi-slice CT can produce high-resolution brain images within one minute. IV contrast agents may be used to show: breakdown of the blood-brain-barrier (BBB), e.g., in tumours and inflammation; and enhanced vascular perfusion, e.g., in AVM. 'Ring' enhancement is typically seen in abscess, metastasis, glioblastomas, and dermoid cysts.

CT is more widely accessible than MRI. The scan time is shorter and therefore more suitable for patients with unstable conditions (e.g., head injury, ICH) and those who are confused and restless. It is more sensitive than MRI for detection of intracranial haemorrhage, calcification (e.g., meningioma), and bone pathology (e.g., fracture).

Magnetic resonance imaging (MRI)

Elements with an odd number of protons or electrons can be induced to resonate when placed in a strong magnetic field. Electromagnetic energy is applied as radiofrequency (RF) pulse, which causes vibration of water protons, releasing a signal to constitute the brain images. Relaxation time is the time taken for protons to return to equilibrium following the RF pulse, and is determined by two processes known as T1 and T2.

T1 weighted image provides good anatomical resolution, e.g., grey-white matter differentiation. The appearance of different structures is listed in Table 2.1. IV gadolinium highlights areas of BBB breakdown.

Table 2.1   T1 weighted image

Appears dark (low signal, long T1)	Appears bright (high signal, short T1)
CSF	lipid
calcium	gadolinium
deoxyhaemoglobin	methaemoglobin
air	melanin
oedema	proteinaceous fluid

T2 weighted image enables detection of increase in cerebral water content (e.g., oedema) which occurs in most neoplastic and inflammatory conditions. The appearance of different structures is listed in Table 2.2. The **FLAIR** (fluid attenuated inversion recovery) sequence produces T2 weighted images with CSF suppression (becoming dark), thus enhancing the sensitivity of detection of periventricular lesions (e.g., plaques, ischaemic areas, hippocampal sclerosis).

Table 2.2   T2 weighted image

Appears dark (low signal, long T2)	Appears bright (high signal, short T2)
bone/calcium	CSF
haemosiderin	liquids
deoxyhaemoglobin	oedema
methaemoglobin	
air	

Diffusion weighted imaging (DWI) sequence is extremely sensitive in detecting acute ischemic lesion (as early as 30 minutes after stroke onset); it is often interpreted together with the **ADC** (apparent diffusion coefficient) map in acute stroke imaging.

Gradient echo sequence is used to detect acute cerebral haemorrhage. It has similar sensitivity as CT.

Diffusor tensor imaging may be used to detect pathology of the pyramidal fibres, e.g., degeneration of corticospinal tract in motor neurone disease.

Perfusion weighted imaging refers to a variety of MRI techniques, e.g., mean transit time and cerebral blood flow to calculate cerebral tissue perfusion, which is very useful before considering revascularization therapy (e.g., in Moyamoya disease).

MR spectroscopy (MRS) determines the concentration of various metabolites in brain tissue, e.g., low N-acetyl-aspartate (NAA) and high choline in high-grade gliomas.

Functional magnetic resonance imaging (fMRI) is used to obtain functional information by visualizing cortical activity. It detects subtle alterations in blood flow in response to various stimuli or actions including speech and motor function. This provides essential information prior to epilepsy surgery.

Phase contrast (PC) MRI can be used to study CSF flow mechanics, e.g., to differentiate communicating from non-communicating hydrocephalus, localize the level of obstruction, and evaluate posterior fossa cystic malformations.

Advantages of MRI

- Multiplanar capacity without ionizing radiation
- Good differentiation among soft tissues and pathological lesion
- Good visualization of structures encased by bone, e.g., posterior fossa, temporal lobe, orbit
- Non-invasive evaluation of vascular anatomy using time of flight (TOF) technique (see MR angiography)
- Gadolinium has far fewer side effects than iodinated contrast. The risk of serious anaphylaxis is less than 0.1%. However, patients with renal failure may develop nephrogenic systemic fibrosis. Premedication with steroids and antihistamines may help alleviate these side effects.

Disadvantages of MRI

- Cardiac pacemakers, with the exception of recent models, are MR incompatible.
- Metallic implants or retained foreign bodies are incompatible with MR scanning, but many recent metal devices are MR compatible.
- Image quality is degraded with restless patients, who may require sedation with benzodiazepines, chloral hydrate or monitored anaesthesia care.
- Claustrophobia in a small proportion of patients ($< 5\%$)
- Long imaging time is partially overcome by newer generation machines.
- Poor visualization of calcified lesions, e.g., tuberculoma
- Artefacts are common and expertise is required for proper interpretation.

Single photon emission computed tomography (SPECT)

It provides measurement of cerebral blood flow, oxygen, and glucose consumption using radioactive ligands, e.g., ^{99}mTc-HMPAO, ^{133}I-iodoamphetamine (IMP). ^{11}C-flumazenil binds to benzodiazepine receptor and may be used to detect areas of neuronal damage. Major applications include evaluation of cerebral perfusion in patients with stroke and demonstration of epileptic focus (increased signal in the ictal and peri-ictal period; reduced signal in the inter-ictal period).

Positron emission tomography (PET)

Short-lived radionuclides (e.g., 11C, 14O, 18F) are generated by a cyclotron which emits positrons after IV administration. Tomographic images of cerebral blood flow, oxygen or glucose consumption are then produced. Specific metabolic processes in the brain can be studied by coupling radioactive tracers with certain biochemical substance (e.g., opiate). Major applications include evaluation of degenerative brain diseases, pre-surgical evaluation of epilepsy (the epileptic focus being hypometabolic), and detection of tumour recurrence and dissemination (as opposed to radiation necrosis and demyelination).

Cerebral vascular imaging

Digital subtraction angiography (DSA)

- Gold standard for detection of cerebral vessel abnormalities
- Catheter angiography: selective catheterization of the carotid and/or vertebral arteries is performed following percutaneous femoral or brachial artery puncture.
- DSA: photographic reversal of the first film superimposed digitally on subsequent angiographic images in order to obtain a subtraction image electronically. This technique produces better delineation of the blood vessels.
- Risks include vessel damage, contrast reaction, renal failure, groin haematoma, and pseudoaneurysm formation. In experienced hands, the overall risk of permanent neurological complications is less than 1%, and transient deficits less than 3%.
- Endovascular procedure is a treatment option for certain vascular lesions, including arterial stenosis/occlusion, aneurysm, AVM, and arteriovenous fistula. Major complications are non-target embolization, arterial thrombosis or dissection, intracranial haemorrhage, and cranial nerve trauma.

CT angiography

Multiple thin slices are obtained within 1 minute following a bolus injection of iodinated contrast. 3-D images of the blood vessels are reconstructed after acquisition of axial source images. It has a high correlation with conventional cerebral angiography and is superior to MRA.

MR angiography (MRA)

MR technique without contrast using time of flight sequence can obtain good visualization of carotid, vertebral, and cerebral vessels, and hence is a useful screening tool in suspected cerebrovascular disease. Administration of contrast gadolinium will provide more anatomical details on structural vascular abnormalities.

Ultrasonography of cerebral arteries

- Ultrasound of the extracranial carotid or vertebral arteries. Regular ultrasound creates a picture from the bounced sound waves at tissue planes; it shows atherosclerotic plaques or blood clots and enables measurement of the intimo-medial thickness. Doppler examines how sound waves are reflected off flowing objects, e.g., RBC. Duplex ultrasound combines Doppler and regular ultrasound; it measures flow velocity and direction and demonstrates occlusion, stenosis, and/or steal phenomenon.
- Transcranial Doppler. It studies the basal segments of the major cerebral arteries by making use of the three natural acoustic windows (temporal, occipital, and orbital) of the skull. It can detect intracranial atherosclerosis, assess vasospasm following SAH, and monitor microembolic signals (for assessment of the risk of recurrent embolism).

Neurophysiology

Nerve conduction study (NCS)

- Percutaneous electrical stimulation of a peripheral nerve excites all the axons within a nerve trunk and the generated impulses are recorded at a distance away from the stimulus. Skin surface electrodes are often used. Needle electrode is sometimes used if the target muscle is very atrophic.
- Potentials recorded from sensory nerve stimulation are of low amplitude (5–50 μV) and averaging can be used to eliminate the background noise.
- The motor unit consists of a single lower motor neuron and the muscle fibres it innervates. Compound muscle action potentials (cMAP) refers to the summation of the motor units of a specific

muscle (e.g., abductor digiti minimi) upon electrical stimulation; its latency, amplitude, and waveform are recorded.

- Motor conduction velocity is 50–60 m/s for the upper limb and 45–50 m/s for the lower limb. This parameter is useful in differentiating demyelinating from axonal neuropathies and in confirming entrapment neuropathy (by presence of conduction block). F-wave study is performed to look for more proximal nerve lesions, e.g., radiculopathies or plexopathies.
- Repetitive nerve stimulation study is often used to evaluate the neuromuscular junction. In patients with MG, at a stimulus rate of 3 Hz, the cMAP shows progressive reduction of amplitude from the 4th or 5th response. A more than 10% decrement in amplitude is considered abnormal and suggestive of MG. Recordings from the proximal muscle groups, e.g., trapezius and facial muscles, are more sensitive in patients with ocular myasthenia. In Eaton-Lambert syndrome, the characteristic feature is progressive increase in cMAP amplitude upon tetanic stimulation (at 20–50 Hz).

Electromyography (EMG)

- Routine concentric needle records the electric potentials generated by about ten muscle fibres at close proximity of the needle tip.
- In normal muscles, the background activity is silent at rest. A few motor unit action potentials (MUAP) are activated at mild volitional activity discharging at 10–20 Hz. The MUAP will overlap to form an interference pattern upon maximum contraction of the muscle.
- Denervation changes (in neuropathic conditions) consist of fibrillations, positive sharp waves and fasciculations at rest (known as spontaneous activity), long duration polyphasic units during volition, and reduced interference pattern on maximum contraction. Giant MUAP may be seen following reinnervation.
- Myopathic changes consist of small spiky or polyphasic units. Early recruitment is observed with mild exertion. Spontaneous

activity may be seen in inflammatory myopathies. In muscular dystrophies, myotonic discharges with dive-bomber sound are present.

- Quantitative EMG requires the use of single fibre or monopolar needle. It determines the fibre density and degree of jittering, and is useful in the diagnosis of ocular MG and certain forms of muscular dystrophies.

Evoked potentials

Evoked potentials are electrical potentials generated by neural structures in response to sensory stimulus. Averaging cuts off the noise and background EEG activity, thereby enhancing the quality of recording. This technique has a high sensitivity for lesion documentation in the sensory pathways.

Visual evoked potentials (VEP)

Black and white checkerboard patterns or stroboscopic flashes are used to activate the occipital visual area. The P_{100} response is widely used to assess the integrity of the central visual pathway. Marked delay of P_{100} is suggestive of demyelination of the anterior visual pathway (e.g., optic neuritis). It is useful for detection of subclinical optic nerve lesions (e.g., retrobulbar optic neuritis in MS) and differentiation between functional and organic blindness. Flash LED goggles are used in children or those who cannot visually fixate on a distant object.

Somatosensory evoked potentials (SEP)

Stimuli are administered to the median, ulnar or posterior tibial nerves and recording electrodes are placed cutaneously at the plexus, spine, and scalp. Potentials are recorded corresponding to sequential activation of the neural structures along the dorsal column. Interpeak latencies are used to estimate the central conduction time, which is often prolonged in patients with spinal cord lesions (e.g., MS, syringomyelia, CSM). Giant SEP are characteristic of certain myoclonic disorders (e.g., progressive myoclonic epilepsy and cortical myoclonus). Intra-operative SEP monitoring is often employed during surgical correction of spinal scoliosis or resection of intramedullary lesions.

Brainstem auditory evoked potentials (BAEP)

The potentials are generated by brainstem auditory pathways following administration of auditory clicks. Five waveforms are usually recognized, but waves I, III, and V are most consistently recorded. The I–III interpeak latency measures conduction from the acoustic nerve to lower pons whereas III–V interpeak latency measures conduction from the rostral pontine to midbrain structure. BAEP is helpful for detection of subclinical brainstem lesions (e.g., MS, central pontine myelinolysis). It is a useful screening procedure for acoustic neuroma and other cerebellopontine angle tumours. It can also be used to assess hearing in infants and kids.

Transcranial magnetic stimulation (TMS)

A round or figure-of-eight coil is applied over the vertex or motor area. The coil produces small electric currents in a small region of the brain under the coil via electromagnetic induction. Surface recordings are made at the hand or lower limb muscles to register the activated cMAP. Single pulse TMS can be used to evaluate the integrity of the motor pathway in stroke, MS, motor neurone disease, head injury, and movement disorders. Repetitive TMS has been used in treatment of drug-resistant major depressive disorder and neuropathic pain, and in stroke rehabilitation.

Electroencephalography (EEG)

- EEG records spontaneous electrical activity of the brain. Activation procedures (e.g., photic stimulation, hyperventilation) are often employed to increase the sensitivity of detecting abnormalities. Small metal discs are attached to the scalp and ear lobes according to the international 10–20 system. Brain activity is amplified a million times and recorded on paper or computer.

- Frequency bands of activity include: delta activity (< 4 Hz), theta activity (4–7 Hz), alpha activity (8–13 Hz), and beta activity (> 13 Hz).

- A normal EEG in an adult during relaxed wakefulness consists of well-formed symmetrical posterior alpha activity, which attenuates upon eye opening. Small amounts of beta activity are often seen at frontal-central regions, and can be accentuated by anxiety or mental arithmetic.

- Hyperventilation for 3 minutes is commonly employed to induce epileptic discharges. Children often develop symmetrical high-amplitude delta waves to hyperventilation, which should not be considered epileptic.

- Photic stimulation delivers repetitive brief flashes of light at a frequency of 1–30 Hz. Photoparoxysmal response (PPR) is characterized by bilateral spike wave or polyspike wave complexes which outlast the stimulus by a few seconds, which is the hallmark of photosensitive epilepsy.

- Sleep EEG is useful for evaluation of nocturnal epilepsy. Sleep deprivation can both facilitate sleep and activate epileptiform discharges.

- Epileptiform discharges consist of spikes, sharp waves, spikes and slow waves, sharp and slow waves, periodic and pseudoperiodic complexes, triphasic waves, and certain fast activities. Their presence supports the diagnosis of epilepsy, but artefacts should first be excluded.

- Video-EEG and ambulatory EEG recordings can be used to capture ictal EEG during an attack. They also help differentiate non-epileptic seizure from epilepsy and identify the epileptic focus during pre-surgical evaluation. Intracranial EEG recordings may produce very useful localizing information in extratemporal epilepsy or those with double pathology.

Polysomnography records selected physiological parameters during sleep: EEG, eye movements, submental EMG, ECG, limb movements, respiration, body position, ear or finger oximetry, and snoring events. Sleep staging is automatically performed by computer software. The following disorders require polysomnogram for proper diagnosis:

- Sleep apnoea syndromes: obstructive, central or mixed
- Narcolepsy, often in conjunction with MSLT
- Idiopathic hypersomnia
- Periodic leg movements
- REM sleep behavioural disorder
- Parasomnia, e.g., sleep walking, night terrors

Multiple sleep latency test (MSLT)

MSLT is designed to evaluate excessive daytime sleepiness. The test consists of five 20-minute naps with each nap 2 hours apart. The onset latency of REM (rapid eye movement) sleep and non-REM sleep is determined for each nap. Normal patients have mean sleep latencies more than 10 minutes and not more than one REM period. Pathologic sleepiness is defined as mean sleep latency of less than 5 minutes. The presence of two or more REM periods is suggestive of narcolepsy, provided that sleep apnoea is excluded by sleep study.

Miscellaneous

Lumbar puncture (LP)

Indications

1. Diagnostic: analysis of the cerebrospinal fluid (CSF) is essential in making the diagnosis of CNS infection, SAH, demyelination, inflammatory and neoplastic disorders, and conditions associated with raised CSF pressure.
2. Therapeutic: removal of CSF in idiopathic intracranial hypertension and normal pressure hydrocephalus; intrathecal administration of cytotoxic drugs in CNS lymphoma and leukaemia; intrathecal baclofen for relief of intractable spinal spasticity (infusion pump is necessary for long-term administration).

Contraindications

1. Raised CSF pressure due to focal brain lesions: LP may lead to coning, which is fatal. CT/MRI brain is obligatory prior to LP. Absence of papilloedema does not guarantee normal CSF pressure.
2. Spinal block
3. Bleeding tendency (e.g., platelet count < 50, INR > 1.5) would incur significant risk of bleeding.
4. Local sepsis (e.g., skin infection, bedsore): risk of introducing meningitis

Complications

1. Headache occurs in 10% of patients and is due to CSF leakage resulting in low pressure. It is more likely with multiple punctures or the use of large gauge needles. Tinnitus or sixth nerve palsies may rarely occur due to downward traction on the brainstem. It is characteristically aggravated by standing up or moving around. IV saline infusion, simple analgesics or caffeine may ameliorate the headache (see also Chapter 5).
2. Rare but serious complications include coning with brainstem compression (e.g., transtentorial), precipitation of aneurysmal SAH, aseptic meningitis, subdural or epidural haematomas, and direct injury to spinal nerve roots, e.g., L4/L5 or cauda equina

Muscle biopsy

- The selected muscle should be moderately weak (power Grade 3/5–4/5) and free from previous trauma (including IMI). Usually the deltoid, biceps or vastus medialis is sampled. The pathologist has to be informed about the clinical problem to maximize the diagnostic yield.
- Muscle biopsy is most helpful in establishing the diagnosis of inflammatory myopathies, muscular dystrophies, and mitochondrial myopathies. Apart from routine haematoxyllin and eosin staining, special tests are available to study specific enzymes or immune markers.

Nerve biopsy

The sural nerve is commonly chosen as little function is lost after it is transected. The indications are mononeuritis multiplex, asymmetric polyneuropathy, or nerves thickening due to unknown aetiology. The microscopic pathology may show: axonal degeneration, demyelination or mixed; vasculitis; deposition of exogenous material (e.g., amyloid); specific pathology (e.g., onion skin in HMSN).

3 Cranial Nerve Disorders

The 12 pairs of cranial nerves (Figure 3.1) innervate most structures of the head and neck. They traverse the meninges, subarachnoid space, bony structures of the cranium, and superficial soft tissues. The cranial nerves may be affected at any site along their course. Bilateral supranuclear innervation is present for all cranial nerves except for the lower facial muscles, trapezius, sternomastoid, and tongue.

Cranial nerve dysfunction may be the presenting complaint of many disorders.

Patterns of involvement

Cranial mononeuropathy

Isolated cranial nerve dysfunction is usually due to a vascular cause (e.g., III nerve palsy in DM), trauma (e.g., IV nerve palsy), or an intrinsic nerve lesion (e.g., Bell's palsy, neurofibroma).

Cranial polyneuropathy

Common causes include:
- Chronic meningitis, e.g., TB, cryptococcus, malignancy. The VI nerve is usually affected first.
- Granulomatous and vasculitic processes, e.g., Wegener's granulomatosis, PAN, cranial arteritis
- Neoplastic, e.g., NPC, carcinomatous or leukaemic/lymphomatous infiltration of meninges, temporal bone meningioma
- Demyelination, e.g., bilateral VII in AIDP; III, IV, and VI in Miller Fisher syndrome

- Cerebello-pontine angle lesion: commonly VIII, V, VII (with ataxia and long tract signs in big lesions)
- Cavernous sinus lesion: III, IV, VI, V (ophthalmic and maxillary divisions) ± II, e.g., Tolosa-Hunt syndrome, cavernous sinus thrombosis
- Raised ICP can cause impaired abduction of both eyes, suggestive of bilateral VI nerve palsy (false localizing sign).
- Idiopathic cranial polyneuropathy (sparing olfactory and auditory nerves)

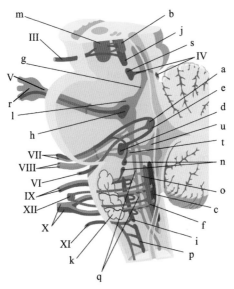

Figure 3.1   A schematic drawing of the brainstem near the mid-sagittal plane showing afferent (red) and efferent (blue) fibres of the cranial nerves (in Roman numbers) with the corresponding nuclei (labelled in alphabets). (a) abducens nucleus; (b) accessory oculomotor (Edinger-Westphal) nucleus; (c) dorsal vagal nucleus; (d) facial nucleus; (e) geniculum of facial nerve; (f) hypoglossal nucleus; (g) mesencephalic nucleus of trigeminal nerve; (h) motor nucleus of trigeminal nerve; (i) nucleus ambiguus; (j) oculomotor nucleus; (k) olive; (l) principal sensory nucleus of trigeminal nerve; (m) red nucleus; (n) rostral (superior) and caudal (inferior) salivatory nuclei; (o) solitary tract nucleus; (p) spinal nucleus of accessory nerve; (q) spinal tract and nucleus of trigeminal nerve.

DISORDERS OF INDIVIDUAL CRANIAL NERVES

Olfactory nerve (I)

The sensory fibres arise from the smell receptors in the nasal mucosa, traverse the cribriform plate and synapse in the olfactory bulb. The postsynaptic fibres form the olfactory tract, which passes to the olfactory cortex in the anteromedial surface of the temporal lobe.

Causes of anosmia

- Upper respiratory infection: most common; transient in the majority, but may be permanent
- Trauma: common
- Tumour, e.g., olfactory groove meningioma
- Congenital anosmia: rare

Optic nerve (II)

The visual pathway (Figure 3.2) starts with the rods and cones at the retina, the fibres of which form the optic nerve. The nasal optic nerve fibres decussate at the optic chiasma whereas the temporal fibres run ipsilaterally. Hence, the optic tract contains the ipsilateral temporal fibres and contralateral nasal fibres. The optic tract ends at the lateral geniculate body, and the visual pathway continues ipsilaterally as the optic radiation to reach the visual cortex of the occipital lobe.

Reduced visual acuity

In optic nerve or chiasma lesions, reduced visual acuity is often preceded by impairment of colour vision. Retinal lesions and lens problems (e.g., refractive errors, keratoconus, and cataract) should be excluded.

Visual field defects

Visual field defects at the different sites along the visual pathway
are shown in Figure 3.2.

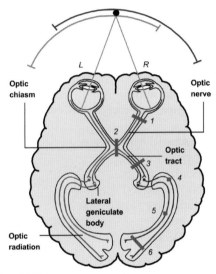

Defects in visual field

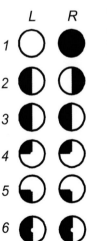

Figure 3.2   A schematic drawing of the visual
pathway illustrating the typical visual field
defects and the corresponding lesion sites.

(1) optic nerve lesion (e.g., optic neuritis):
monocular amaurosis

(2) optic chiasma lesion (e.g., pituitary macroadenoma): bitemporal hemianopia

(3) optic tract lesion (e.g., craniopharyngioma):
incongruent homonymous hemianopia

(4) temporal optic radiation lesion (e.g., post-
temporal lobectomy): homonymous upper
quadrantic hemianopia

(5) parietal optic radiation lesion (e.g., parietal
glioma): homonymous lower quadrantic
hemianopia

(6) visual cortical lesion (e.g., occipital lobe
infarct): dense homonymous hemianopia
with macular sparing.

Papilloedema (Figure 3.3c)

This term refers to swelling and erythema of the optic discs with blurred margins. In patients with raised intracranial pressure (ICP), the blind spot is enlarged and the retinal veins are engorged and non-pulsatile at the early stage. When advanced, retinal haemorrhages appear around the disc. Transient visual blurring is due to reduced optic nerve perfusion and may precede blindness.

Common causes include:
- Raised ICP
  - Intracranial mass lesions
  - Cerebral oedema, e.g., encephalitis, cerebral infarction
  - SAH
  - Benign intracranial hypertension
- Accelerated hypertension
- Optic disc disorder
  - Retinal vein occlusion (Figure 3.3f)
  - Disc infiltration, e.g., leukaemia
- Metabolic causes
  - Carbon dioxide retention
  - Chronic hypoxia

Optic neuropathy

Unilateral optic neuropathy may be caused by:
- Optic nerve compression, e.g., orbital meningioma
- Optic nerve tumour
- Ischaemic optic neuropathy
- Unilateral optic neuritis, e.g., SLE, NMOSD, MS

Bilateral optic neuropathy may result from:
- Hereditary optic atrophy, e.g., Leber's disease
- Malnutrition, e.g., vitamin A and B_{12} deficiency
- Drugs, e.g., ethambutol
- Toxic substance, e.g., methanol, n-hexane, lead
- Bilateral optic neuritis, e.g., SLE, NMOSD, MS

Retrobulbar neuritis:
The fundal appearance is normal because the inflammatory process is behind the eyeball. It is usually due to demyelinating disease

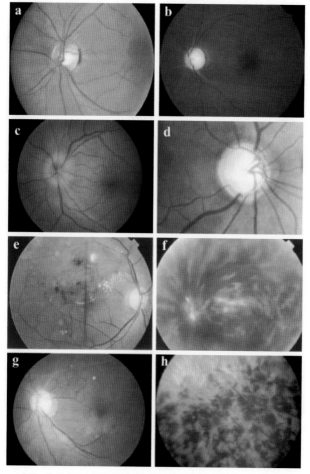

Figure 3.3 Colour plates of fundi showing (a) a normal fundus, (b) optic atrophy, (c) early papilloedema, (d) glaucoma, (e) superior temporal branch retinal artery occlusion, (f) central retinal vein occlusion, (g) superior temporal branch retinal artery occlusion with narrow arteries, tortuous veins plus disc pallor, and (h) retinitis pigmentosa.

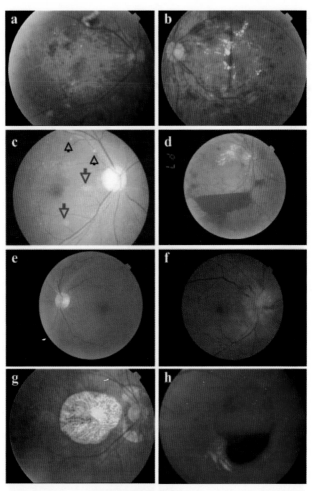

Figure 3.4   Colour plates of fundi showing (a) background diabetic retinopathy with hard exudates plus dot and blot haemorrhages, (b) exudative maculopathy plus background diabetic retinopathy, (c) two cholesterol emboli (black arrows) in the superior temporal branch of the retinal artery, soft exudates (blue arrows), arteriosclerosis plus disc pallor, (d) DM fundi with proliferative changes, dot and blot hemorrhages, post-laser scars, subhyaloid hemorrhage and hard exudate, (e) grade II hypertensive fundus, (f) grade IV hypertensive fundus, (g) disciform macular scar, and (h) sub-hyaloid haemorrhage.

(e.g., MS) and may be unilateral or bilateral. Subclinical forms can be detected by marked prolongation of the P_{100} latency on VEP.

Optic atrophy (Figure 3.3b)

The optic disc is pale with distinct margins; the causes are those of optic neuropathy. Secondary optic atrophy may arise as a sequel of long-standing papilloedema.

Pupil disorders

Sympathetic fibres to the eye originate in the hypothalamus and descend via the brainstem to the superior cervical ganglion at T1 level. The post-synaptic fibres form a plexus surrounding the internal carotid artery and proceed to the pupil in the nasociliary nerves. They are responsible for pupillary dilation. In contrast, parasympathetic fibres pass from the ciliary ganglion in the short ciliary nerve to the pupil constrictor muscles.

The light reflex arc is mediated by afferent fibres in the optic nerve; these fibres reach both lateral geniculate bodies and are relayed to the Edinger-Westphal nuclei. Efferent fibres then pass via the III nerve to the ciliary ganglion and the pupil. Fibres responsible for the convergence reflex relay from the convergence centre to both geniculate bodies. The efferent fibres then pass to the Edinger-Westphal nucleus, ciliary ganglion, and pupils.

The causes of pupil abnormalities can be deduced from the pupillary size and reaction to light (Table 3.1).

Argyll Robertson pupil

It is ascribed to damage in the periaqueductal area. The typical pupil is small, irregular, fixed to light but reacts to accommodation. Causes include meningovascular syphilis, DM, and brainstem encephalitis.

Table 3.1   Common causes of pupillary abnormalities

Reaction to light	Small pupils	Large pupils
Non-reactive	Argyll Robertson pupil (often irregular)	Holmes-Adie pupil
	Pontine haemorrhage	Post-traumatic iridoplegia
	Opiates	Mydriatic drops
	Pilocarpine eye drops	Oculomotor palsy
	Atropine effect	Ciliary ganglionitis
	Synechiae	
Reactive	Senile miosis	Physiological anisocoria
	Horner's syndrome	Anxiety

Holmes-Adie pupil

This is an idiopathic condition often associated with loss of knee jerks and impairment of sweating. The typical pupil is widely dilated. It reacts very slowly to light but briskly to miotics. It is usually unilateral (80%) and more often found in women.

Horner's syndrome

The typical features include miosis, enophthalmos, ptosis, and reduced sweating on the ipsilateral side of the face. It is due to disruption of the sympathetic fibres, which may occur at different sites.
- Hemisphere, e.g., massive infarction
- Brainstem, e.g., vascular lesions, tumour, demyelination
- Cervical spinal cord, e.g., syringomyelia, cord gliomas
- T1 root, e.g., Pancoast's tumour, degenerative disc disease
- Sympathetic chain, e.g., neck surgery

Oculomotor, trochlear, and abducens nerves (III, IV, VI)

These nerves supply the extraocular muscles and control eye movements. The superior oblique muscle is supplied by the IV nerve, the lateral rectus by the VI, and the rest by the III. The III nerve also supplies the levator palpebrae superioris and carries parasympathetic fibres responsible for pupil constriction.

Oculomotor (III) nerve

The nucleus of the III nerve lies in the central part of the midbrain. It emerges between the cerebral peduncles, enters the cavernous sinus, and passes to the orbit through the superior orbital fissure. A severe lesion causes complete ptosis. Diplopia occurs in all directions except on lateral gaze to the side of the lesion, and the eye is deviated outwards and downwards.

An isolated III nerve lesion is often due to ischaemia, in which case the pupil is not affected and the ptosis commonly partial. It may also be compressed by a posterior communicating artery aneurysm or a tumour. Because the parasympathetic fibres are situated at the outermost layer of the nerve and therefore liable to be compressed, the pupil becomes dilated and non-reactive.

Trochlear (IV) nerve

Its nucleus lies at the dorsum of the midbrain. The nerve passes through the posterior fossa, cavernous sinus, and superior orbital fissure before ending in the superior oblique muscle. This muscle pulls the eye downwards when it is at the adducted position.

An isolated lesion is usually congenital, post-traumatic, or secondary to DM. The affected eye rotates slightly outwards with a compensatory head tilts towards the unaffected side. Maximum diplopia occurs on looking downwards and inwards, posing difficulty in descending stairs.

In the presence of a III nerve lesion, the IV nerve is tested by asking the patient to look downwards. An intact IV nerve is present if there is depression, with or without intorsion of the eyeball.

Abducens (VI) nerve

The nucleus lies in the lower pons and its fibres emerge from the brainstem at the pontomedullary junction. It then enters the cavernous sinus and passes to the orbit. A VI nerve lesion is characterized by impaired abduction of the eye.

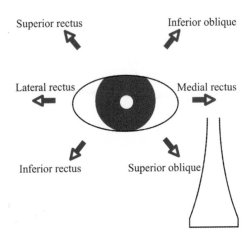

Figure 3.5 A schematic drawing of the right eye with the arrows showing the direction of pulling of the individual extraocular muscle on the eye.

An isolated lesion may be due to trauma, ischaemia or raised ICP.

Approach to diplopia

Binocular diplopia is due to any lesion which prevents conjugate eye movements, e.g., displaced eyeball, MG, ocular myopathy, or a lesion of the III, IV or VI nerve.

In order to determine which cranial nerve is involved, it is necessary to determine in what direction of gaze the diplopia is maximum. Maximum diplopia occurs in the direction of the weak extraocular muscle. Ask the patient to look at each side and then up and down. The false image that arises from the affected eye is more peripheral and less distinct. It disappears when the affected eye is covered.

Nystagmus

Nystagmus is an involuntary biphasic rhythmic ocular oscillation in which one or both phases are slow. The nystagmus direction is defined as the direction of the fast component which is easily observed and may be horizontal, vertical, diagonal, or rotational.

Nystagmus is tested first with the eyes fixated on a distant object and then with the eyes moving from side to side. Nystagmus or nystagmoid jerks may be encountered in normal subjects when the eyeball reaches extreme positions. It is only significant when it persists after the eyeballs shift to a new position. The fast phase (saccadic) returns the eyes to the target position and the slow phase drifts the eyes towards the central position (pathological component). The fast component is not observed in pendular nystagmus in which oscillations are of equal velocity.

Three grades of nystagmus are recognized:
Grade I: nystagmus present in one direction of gaze
Grade II: nystagmus present in primary position
Grade III: nystagmus in all directions of gaze

Nystagmus may result from dysfunction of the vestibular end-organ, vestibular nerve, brainstem or cerebellum. The commonly encountered nystagmus are:
- Congenital nystagmus
  - present from birth throughout life
  - associated with albinism
  - usually binocular, horizontal, and pendular
  - aggravated by visual fixation
  - patient unaware of nystagmus
- Acquired pendular nystagmus
  - associated with brainstem or cerebellar lesions, e.g., MS
  - usually horizontal
- Vestibular nystagmus
  - usually Grade II and due to dysfunction of vestibular end-organ or its connections
- Gaze-evoked nystagmus
  - the most common form of nystagmus
  - usually horizontal ± torsional jerk nystagmus
  - often due to adverse effect of drugs (e.g., phenytoin, alcohol, barbiturates, benzodiazepines), but may be due to brainstem or cerebellar lesion

- Upbeat nystagmus
  - occurs in primary position
  - may be due to brainstem lesion, e.g., MS, cerebellar degeneration
- Downbeat nystagmus
  - occurs in primary position
  - accentuated by lateral gaze, downgaze, and convergence
  - present in Arnold-Chiari malformation and cerebellar degeneration

Trigeminal nerve (V)

It is predominantly a sensory nerve. Sensory fibres carrying light touch sensation enter the nucleus in the pons, while those fibres carrying pain and temperature sensations enter from the spinal tract of the V nerve and end in the spinal nucleus in the medulla. Motor fibres arise in the upper pons and supply the muscles of mastication (masseters, pterygoids, and temporalis).

Lesions of trigeminal nerve may occur at different levels:
- Middle cranial fossa, e.g., tumour, aneurysm
- Brainstem: intrinsic lesions, e.g., tumour, ischaemia, demyelination; extrinsic lesions, e.g., acoustic neuroma, meningioma, neurofibroma
- Skull base, e.g., metastatic tumour, chronic meningitis
- Extracranial course, e.g, trauma, vasculitis, leprosy

Trigeminal neuralgia

This idiopathic condition is characterized by intense paroxysmal pain confined to the distribution of the V nerve. It usually occurs in middle-aged subjects. If it arises in younger patients, secondary trigeminal pain has to be considered.

It is unilateral in most cases and usually involves one or two adjacent branches of the nerve, commonly the maxillary and mandibular divisions. Each attack usually lasts for a few seconds to one minute. Trigger spots may be identified at the lips, chin, gum or tongue. During an attack, the patient may have his face screwed up in agony (*tic douloureux*). Spontaneous remission may last for several months or years in the early stages.

It is diagnosed by the typical history and normal physical examination. If there are sensory or motor signs, secondary causes, e.g., cerebello-pontine angle tumour, should be considered.

The majority of patients respond to carbamazepine. Gabapentin, pregabalin, phenytoin, and baclofen may be added if necessary. Amitriptyline is also used in severe cases.

When medical therapy fails, posterior craniectomy with microvascular decompression of the trigeminal nerve (with or without highly selective rhizotomy) is an effective treatment with low morbidity and low recurrence. Other forms of surgical intervention such as thermocoagulation of the ganglion or section of the sensory root are also effective, but are associated with a higher complication rate. Radiosurgery, e.g., gamma-knife, is effective in some cases, with the advantage of being non-invasive.

Facial nerve (VII)

The nerve nucleus lies in the pons. After emerging from the brainstem, its fibres enter the internal auditory meatus, pass through the facial canal, and leave the skull through the stylomastoid foramen.

Two types of facial palsy, viz. UMN and LMN, should be distinguished. UMN facial palsy results from a lesion of the corticobulbar pathway. It commonly presents with contralateral lower facial weakness; the upper face is minimally or not affected because of bilateral corticobulbar innervation.

LMN facial palsy (facial nerve palsy) results from a lesion in the nucleus or trunk of the facial nerve. It manifests as ipsilateral upper and lower facial palsy with or without loss of taste sensation of the anterior two-third of the tongue. Hyperacusis may be present if the lesion is proximal.

Common causes of facial nerve lesion include:
- Idiopathic (Bell's palsy): most common
- Infection: Ramsay-Hunt syndrome, Lyme disease
- Demyelination: AIDP

- Granulomatous: TBM
- Neoplastic: cerebello-pontine angle tumour, e.g., acoustic neuroma, malignant infiltration

Bell's palsy

Facial paralysis in this condition is unilateral in most cases, and may occur at any time from infancy to old age. The major cause is presumed to be a viral infection. Nerve ischaemia is implicated in a minority of cases, e.g., due to DM. In the acute stage, the segment of the facial nerve within the canal is swollen, resulting in conduction block with or without nerve fibre damage. Taste disturbance and hyperacusis may be associated features.

The paralysis is usually maximum in 1–2 days. Most patients (85%) recover completely in weeks or months while 15% have residual weakness. A favourable sign is an incomplete palsy in the first week.

A short course of steroids administered at the acute stage expedites recovery. Complications following Bell's palsy include exposure keratitis, residual facial asymmetry, and aberrant reinnervation resulting in hemifacial spasm and crocodile tears. Recurrence takes place in about 5% of patients.

Vestibulocochlear nerve (VIII)

This nerve contains fibres of the cochlear division responsible for hearing and fibres of the vestibular division responsible for balance.

Vertigo

This is a feeling of spinning movement of the subject or the surroundings. It may be due to central or peripheral causes.

Central lesions at the brainstem usually give rise to horizontal nystagmus more prominent towards the side of the lesion. Rotatory and vertical nystagmus may also occur. The nystagmus is usually sustained and non-adaptive.

Common causes of central vertigo include:

- Acute posterior fossa lesions, e.g., brainstem ischaemia
- Cerebello-pontine lesions, e.g., acoustic neuroma
- MS

Peripheral lesions in the inner ear may bring about horizontal nystagmus more prominent away from the side of the lesion. It is usually unsustained and adaptive, and may be dependent on position.

Common causes of peripheral vertigo include:

- Meniere's disease
- Benign paroxysmal positional vertigo
- Vestibular neuronitis
- Drugs and toxic substances, e.g., aminoglycosides, alcohol
- Vestibular migraine

Deafness

Deafness may be due to conductive or sensorineural lesions (Table 3.2). In conductive deafness, bone conduction is better than air conduction, and the patient is not completely deaf. In unilateral sensorineural deafness, air conduction is better than bone conduction and in Weber's test, sound is localized to the normal ear.

Table 3.2   Common causes of deafness

Conductive deafness
Earwax
Trauma, e.g., ruptured tympanic membrane
Infection, e.g., otitis media
Otosclerosis

Sensorineural deafness
Congenital, e.g., congenital rubella
Hereditary, e.g., Alport's syndrome
Drug, e.g., aminoglycosides
Tumour, e.g., acoustic neuroma
Infection, e.g., bacterial meningitis
Vascular, e.g., brainstem ischaemia
Degenerative, e.g., Meniere's disease

Meniere's disease

This condition is characterized by the triad of progressive deafness, tinnitus, and recurrent vertigo. It usually develops in middle-aged subjects with males and females being equally affected.

The pathogenesis is believed to be due to damage to the receptor cells of the cochlea and disturbance of the vestibular system by excessive accumulation of endolymph. It may progress to total sensorineural deafness.

Glossopharyngeal, vagus, and accessory nerves (IX, X, XI)

The IX nerve mediates the taste sense at the posterior one-third of the tongue and pharyngeal sensation. Its motor fibres supply the stylopharyngeus muscle.

The X nerve supplies the pharyngeal and laryngeal muscles and mediates sensation from the larynx.

The XI nerve supplies the sternomastoid and the cranial one-third of the trapezius.

These nerves arise in the lower brainstem and run on the surface of the brainstem in close proximity. They emerge from the skull base through the jugular foramen. Mixed nerve lesions (IX, X, XI) are therefore common, e.g., jugular foramen syndrome.

Pseudobulbar palsy

Pseudobulbar palsy is due to bilateral UMN lesion of the corticobulbar tract. It manifests with a spastic tongue and pharyngeal wall, preservation of the gag reflex, and an exaggerated jaw jerk.

Bulbar palsy

This LMN lesion produces weakness of the pharyngeal wall. Lesions may arise at different sites:

Skull base: tumour, e.g., NPC, meningioma
               infection, e.g., TBM
               malignancy, e.g., carcinomatous meningitis
               vascular, e.g., internal carotid artery aneurysm

Brainstem: tumour, e.g., glioma
               vascular, e.g., infarction
               demyelination
               MND
               syringobulbia

The vagus nerve may also be involved at the neck, e.g., neck surgery, trauma. The left recurrent laryngeal nerve is more often affected than the right because it winds around the ascending aorta. The causes include aortic aneurysm, enlarged left atrium, and carcinoma of lung.

Hypoglossal nerve (XII)

This motor nerve arises in the medulla and leaves the skull through the anterior condylar foramen; it innervates the ipsilateral tongue muscles.

In UMN lesion of the tongue, the muscle bulk is normal. Bilateral UMN lesion produces a spastic tongue with difficulty in protrusion. Causes include brainstem tumour, vascular lesions (e.g., medial medullary syndrome), and MND. Unilateral UMN lesion produces tongue deviation to contralateral side; this is commonly seen in stroke patients with hemiparesis.

LMN lesion gives rise to weakness, wasting, and fasciculations of the tongue. When protruded, the tongue deviates towards the affected side. Common causes include skull base tumours, basal meningitis, neck trauma, and MND.

4 Headache

Headache or cephalalgia is pain felt over the head or face. It is one of the most common types of pain in both sexes and at all ages. Eighty percent of the general population would have experienced one or more episodes within the preceding 3 years. Headache may result in significant morbidity and economic loss. Many sufferers, however, do not consult their doctors, and the use of over-the-counter drugs is very common.

Primary headaches are benign, as are recurrent headaches which do not arise from structural brain lesions; common examples of the latter are tension headache, migraine, and cluster headache. Secondary headaches occur as a symptom of an underlying disease; examples are infection, head injury, vascular disorders, intracranial bleeding, and brain tumours. About 90% of all headaches are primary headaches; these can be effectively managed by family physicians. They can also identify patients who need further investigation and prompt referral to specialists.

Headache is due to pressure, traction, displacement or inflammation of nociceptors with signals traversing the ascending serotoninergic system to reach the midbrain raphe region. Pain-sensitive structures in the head and neck are the scalp and skin, muscles, venous sinuses, meninges, cerebral arteries and veins, nerves and periosteum. The skull, brain parenchyma, and ventricular ependyma are insensitive to pain.

Approach to diagnosis

A detailed and focused history can often establish the diagnosis in a patient with headache (Table 4.1). Useful information includes features of the headache (onset, course, site, radiation, character,

Table 4.1   Differential diagnosis

Character of headache	Possible causes
Acute severe headache	
• With neck rigidity	SAH
	Meningitis or encephalitis
	Systemic infection (meningism)
• Without neck rigidity	Pressor response
	(e.g., phaeochromocytoma)
	Acute glaucoma
	Acute obstructive hydrocephalus
	Expanding intracranial aneurysm
	Carotid or vertebral artery dissection
	ICH
	Head trauma and complications
	Migraine
	Occipital neuralgia
Subacute onset of headache	Expanding intracranial lesion (e.g. subdural haematoma, tumour)
	Progressive hydrocephalus
	Cranial arteritis (age > 50)
	Local infiltration by tumour (e.g., NPC)
	Benign intracranial hypertension
	Sphenoid sinusitis or periorbital cellulitis
	Optic neuritis
	Cerebral vasculitis
	Cerebral venous thrombosis
	CSF hypotension
Recurrent discrete episodes of headache or facial pain	Migraine
	Cluster headache
	Paroxysmal hemicrania
	Trigeminal neuralgia
	Paroxysmal hypertension (e.g., phaeochromocytoma)
	Tolosa-Hunt syndrome
	Benign cough or exertional headache
	Post-herpetic neuralgia

intensity, frequency, duration, triggering or aggravating factor, relieving measures), associated neurological or other physical symptoms, treatment history, family history, sleep pattern, and occupation and emotional profile. A full neurological examination, as well as examination of the BP, skull, cervical spine, teeth, throat, nasal sinuses, eyes and ears, are mandatory. A sound clinical diagnosis would allow the clinician to avoid unnecessary investigations and inappropriate treatment. *The International Classification of Headache Disorders* (third edition, 2013) provides a detailed hierarchical classification of all headache-related disorders.

Investigations and specialist referral

A small proportion of patients require investigations (Table 4.2) and/or specialist referral (Table 4.3), particularly those with features indicating serious diseases.

Principles of treatment

Preventive (prophylactic) therapy with regular medication is indicated for frequent or disabling attacks. Avoidance of triggering factors can be an effective way of prevention. Symptomatic (abortive) therapy is useful for acute attacks.

Table 4.2   Investigations

Investigations	Comments
CBC, ESR, LFT, RFT	To detect systemic diseases ESR markedly raised in cranial arteritis
Plain X-ray	Skull X-ray rarely required unless bony lesion suspected CXR for lung tumour if intracranial metastasis suspected Cervical X-ray for neck or occipital pain
CT/MRI brain	Indicated if persistent or progressive neurological deficits, orbital bruits or focal seizures are present
Cerebral angiography or MRA	To detect arterial dissection, aneurysm, AVM, vasculitis or arterial supply of tumours
CSF pressure and analysis	Prior CT brain advisable since ICP may be raised To document ICP To detect intracranial infection, inflammation or infiltration
ENT evaluation	When suspecting NPC or other ENT causes of headache

Table 4.3   Specialist referral

Referral indicated	Comments
Features of potentially serious disease	Sudden onset of new, severe headache Progressively worsening headache Onset of headache after exertion, straining, coughing or sexual activity Changes in cognitive state Focal neurological signs Systemic features such as fever, arthralgia or myalgia Onset after the age of 50 years
Failure to respond to adequate doses of appropriate medication	Check drug compliance Review diagnosis
Possibility of medication abuse and psychological disturbance	Rebound headache Drug dependence state
Co-morbid conditions complicating drug prescription	Side effects of drugs
Possibility of psychiatric disease	Anxiety neurosis or hypochondriasis
Specialist's reassurance	Anxious patient and/or relatives

SELECTED ENTITIES

Migraine

About 12% of the population experience migraine at some time of their lifetime. The precise mechanism of migraine is uncertain. Recent evidence suggests an important role for the trigeminal vascular system and the neurotransmitter serotonin (5-hydroxy-tryptamine, or 5HT). Changes in the internal or external environment lead to intra- and extra-cranial vascular reactions which, in turn, produce the migrainous headache.

Clinical features

Females are affected more often than males. The onset is usually in the second or third decade. Four phases are recognized:

(1) Prodrome – mental and mood changes, fatigue, or autonomic symptoms for hours to days before headache

(2) Aura – transient focal neurological symptoms usually before headache but sometimes during or after headache; gradual onset, fully reversible, both positive and negative features; lasts 5–60 minutes
   - Homonymous visual: fortification spectra, zigzag lines, flashing lights (positive); scotoma (negative); most common
   - Unilateral sensory: pins and needles (positive); numbness (negative)
   - Dysphasic speech disturbance
   - Associated with depressed regional cerebral blood flow

(3) Headache – episodes of unilateral or bilateral, pulsatile or throbbing, occipital-nuchal or temporal pain of moderate to severe intensity lasting 4–72 hours and associated with nausea, vomiting, diarrhoea, photophobia and phonophobia; aggravation by routine physical activities

(4) Postdrome – a hangover-like state with irritability, listlessness, impaired concentration, fatigue and/or muscle aches lasting up to 24 hours

Precipitating factors may be present:
- Hormonal – menstruation, pregnancy, childbirth, oral contraceptives, menopause
- Emotional – stress, anger, excitement
- Personal or behavioural – change in sleep, irregular meals
- Dietary – starvation, foods containing tyramine, nitrites, sulphites, caffeine, monosodium glutamate or aspartame, citrus fruits, yeast products, dairy products, chocolate, nuts, beer, red wine
- Others – certain drugs, smoking, fluorescent lights, weather changes

Types

- Migraine without aura (in about 75% of patients):
  - Previously known as common migraine or hemicrania simplex
  - ≥ 5 attacks of migraine headache without aura (probable migraine if < 5 attacks)
  - Subtyped according to menstrual relationship: pure menstrual, menstrually related or non-menstrual migraine without aura
- Migraine with aura (in about 20% of patients):
  - Previously known as classic or classical migraine
  - ≥ 2 attacks of migraine headache with aura
  - Previously also named according to the predominate form of aura: ophthalmic, hemiparesthetic, hemiplegic or aphasic migraine, complicated migraine
  - Subtyped according to headache features: typical aura with migraine or non-migraine headache, or typical aura without headache (migraine equivalent or acephalgic migraine)
  - Hemiplegic migraine if aura including motor weakness: familial (the calcium channel genes located in chromosome 19 and 1; male predominant) or sporadic
  - Basilar-type migraine if aura symptoms from the vertebrobasilar territory: dysarthria, vertigo, tinnitus, hypoacusis, diplopia, bilateral visual field symptoms, ataxia, reduced consciousness, bilateral paraesthesia
- Migraine variants:
  - Childhood periodic syndromes: cyclical vomiting, abdominal migraine, benign paroxysmal vertigo
  - Retinal migraine: repeated attacks of migraine headache with monocular visual symptoms, e.g., scintillation, scotoma, blindness
- Migraine complications:
  - Chronic migraine if occurring ≥ 15 days per month for > 3 months; no medication overuse
  - Status migrainosus for a debilitating migraine attack lasting for > 72 hours

- Persistent aura without infarction if aura symptoms lasting for > 1 week
- Migrainous infarction if aura symptoms lasting for > 1 hour plus ischaemic infarction on CT or MRI (see Chapter 6)
- Migraine-triggered seizure if an epileptic seizure occurs during or within 1 hour of aura

Management

Treatment depends on the frequency, intensity, and duration of the headache. Symptomatic treatment is most useful when the attacks are short-lived and infrequent. Preventive therapy is needed in patients with frequent (more than twice per month) or disabling attacks or when symptomatic therapy fails.

- Symptomatic treatment
  - Oral paracetamol or non-steroidal anti-inflammatory drugs (NSAIDs) plus metoclopramide
  - Ergotamine preparations are effective in relieving acute attacks only and should not be used on a regular basis. Excessive use may induce vasospastic symptoms such as pain and paraesthesia in the extremities or cause ergot dependency and rebound headache. Side effects include nausea, and coronary or peripheral ischaemia. Concomitant use with ß-blockers, oral contraceptives or triptans should be avoided. Ergotamine is contraindicated in patients with ischaemic or thyrotoxic heart disease, peripheral vascular disease, or uncontrolled hypertension.
  - Triptans (e.g., sumatriptan 25–100 mg orally or 6 mg sub-cutaneously, naratriptan orally, or zolmitriptan orally) are $5\text{-HT}_{1B/1D}$ agonists that selectively constrict cerebral and dural blood vessels. Side effects include dizziness, somnolence, asthenia, nausea, and tightness and pressure in the throat, neck, and chest. They are contraindicated in patients with ischaemic heart disease, stroke, coronary artery disease, or uncontrolled hypertension. Concomitant use with ergotamine or other triptans should be avoided.

- Status migranosus may require in-patient therapy. Referral to a specialist is recommended.
- Avoid medications during pregnancy. Use paracetamol and/ or opioids when necessary. Nausea and vomiting can be relieved by anti-emetics.
- Preventive therapy
  - Avoid precipitating factors; observe contraindications of medications.
  - Consider prophylactic NSAIDs in menstrual or orgasmic migraine.
  - ß-blockers (e.g., propranolol, atenolol) should be continued for at least 1 month before assessment of efficacy.
  - Calcium channel blockers, e.g., flunarizine, amlodipine
  - Tricyclics, e.g., amitriptyline
  - AEDs, e.g., sodium valproate, gabapentin, phenytoin, topiramate, levetiracetam
  - $5-HT_2$ antagonists, e.g., pizotifen
  - Avoid preventive medications during pregnancy, but ß-blockers and amitriptyline have been used.
  - Botulinum toxin given as multiple injections by trained specialists around the head and neck at 12-week intervals is effective treatment for refractory cases.

Cluster headache

Cluster headache, also known as migrainous neuralgia, is caused by paroxysmal discharges of the central trigeminal and parasympathetic pathways and is associated with dilatation of proximal branches of the internal carotid artery including the ophthalmic artery. It is uncommon but should be considered in patients presenting with appropriate clinical features.

Clinical features

This is a severe unilateral peri- or retro-orbital headache that typically occurs in middle-aged men (males to females = 10 to 1) who are smokers and chronic drinkers. Attacks of headaches tend to occur on a daily basis over weeks to months at a time. Each attack of headache lasts from minutes to hours. It may wake up the patient from sleep. Alcohol and glyceryl trinitrate (a useful diagnostic test) may induce an attack. Nausea, photophobia or aura is absent. Associated symptoms include ipsilateral nasal and ocular congestion, lacrimation, rhinorrhoea, sweating over the forehead and face, and eyelid oedema. About 30–50% of patients develop Horner's syndrome.

Differential diagnosis includes:
- Paroxysmal hemicrania
- Vascular lesion, e.g., carotid dissection, cerebral AVM, vertebral artery aneurysm, cavernous carotid artery aneurysm
- Tumour of brainstem or at occipito-cervical junction
- Inflammatory lesion, e.g., cranial arteritis, Tolosa-Hunt syndrome
- Orbital disease
- Sinusitis
- Trigeminal neuralgia

Treatment

- For acute attacks
  - 100% oxygen therapy for 10 minutes
  - Triptans
  - IM or IV dihydroergotamine
  - A short course of oral prednisolone often takes hours to begin to work and may be used to induce remission.
- Preventive therapy
  - Verapamil
  - Lithium
  - Gabapentin

Paroxysmal hemicrania

This is an uncommon headache syndrome characterized by brief episodes of unilateral pain lasting 2–45 minutes usually over the orbital and temporal regions. Multiple attacks in a single day are typical; some patients have 40–50 attacks within a 24-hour period. Associated autonomic dysfunction such as conjunctival injection, lacrimation, nasal congestion, ptosis, and eyelid oedema is common. Cluster headache is the principal differential diagnosis; paroxysmal hemicrania is more common in females, shorter in duration, and responsive to indomethacin but not oxygen. Many patients may also respond to verapamil, acetazolamide or other NSAIDs.

Tension headache

This is the most common form of benign headache and affects 30–80% of the general population. It is also known as muscle contraction, psychomyogenic, stress, ordinary, essential or idiopathic headache. The headache is diffuse and usually described as mild or moderate 'pressure' or 'tightness' all over the head. It may occur daily and is worse towards the end of the day. Underlying stress, anxiety or depression is often present.

Simple analgesics and muscle relaxants are effective for relief of headache, but drug dependence and rebound headache may develop. Concomitant anxiety or depression should be looked for and treated with counselling, relaxation therapy, and/or judicious use of sedatives or antidepressants. Psychiatric referral may be required in certain cases.

Cranial arteritis

This is also known as temporal arteritis or giant cell arteritis. The underlying pathology is subacute granulomatous inflammation of medium and large arteries with infiltration of lymphocytes, plasma cells, neutrophils and giant cells, and thrombosis may occur in the affected arteries. Typically, a patient aged over 50 has insidious onset of intense headache with non-specific symptoms of malaise, fever and anorexia. Scalp tenderness and jaw claudication may develop. Retinal or optic nerve ischaemia may result in sudden blindness in 25% of untreated cases, and cerebral ischaemia may also occur. Polymyalgia rheumatica (pain and stiffness over the shoulder and pelvic girdle muscles) coexists in about 50% of cases.

ESR is raised. Temporal artery biopsy may reveal thickened arterial wall (often with thrombosis) with giant cell infiltration in the media. However, as the disease process is patchy, the biopsy may be negative.

Once the clinical diagnosis is made, high dose oral prednisolone (45–60 mg daily for several weeks) should be started without awaiting histological confirmation. The steroid dosage may be gradually reduced to 10–20 mg daily and maintained for several months to several years according to the clinical response and ESR.

5 Disorders of Cerebrospinal Fluid Dynamics

The normal CSF pressure is 6–18 cm water in adults and 3–6 cm water in children. The CSF volume ranges from 70–160 ml. About 500 ml of CSF is produced each day by the choroid plexus of the lateral, third, and fourth ventricles, and circulates to the subarachnoid space via the foramina of Magendie and Lushka of the fourth ventricle. It is then reabsorbed through the arachnoid villi into the dural venous sinuses and cerebral veins.

A variety of disorders are caused by abnormally low or high intracranial pressure (ICP).

Raised intracranial pressure

Raised ICP may present with diffuse headache, nausea, vomiting, visual blurring (due to papilloedema), photophobia, blindness (tunnel vision), double vision (false localizing sign of VI nerve palsy), unequal pupils (due to pupil dilation), and impaired consciousness. Symptoms are worsened by coughing, straining, sneezing or lying supine. Acute severe elevation of ICP can lead to bradycardia, hypertension or hypotension, and respiratory impairment. Findings on CT or MRI brain aid the diagnosis of raised ICP and its cause. ICP can be measured via LP or ventriculostomy.

Causes

- Increased brain volume: cerebral oedema, encephalitis
- Mass lesion: tumour, intracerebral haemorrhage, subdural or epidural haematoma, brain abscess, granulomas, parasitic cysts

- Increased CSF volume: obstructive (e.g., aqueductal stenosis, Arnold-Chiari malformation) or communicating hydrocephalus (post-meningitis or SAH)
- Increased blood volume: vasodilatation in CO_2 retention (chronic respiratory failure), malignant hypertension
- Others: benign intracranial hypertension, cranial synostosis, pachymeningitis, breakdown of BBB

Management

- LP is in general contraindicated in patients with raised ICP because of the risk of coning (herniation of the cerebellar tonsils through the foramen magnum). For those with a normal brain scan and raised CSF pressure, the LP needle should be withdrawn once CSF collection is completed for diagnostic analysis. Mannitol may be given concomitantly to lower ICP and reduce risk of herniation.
- The underlying cause should be treated.
- Raised ICP can be controlled using the following measures:
  - Reduce cerebral oedema using hyperosmolar agent (e.g., mannitol, hypertonic saline)
  - Fluid restriction to half of daily requirements
  - Controlled mechanical hyperventilation to induce cerebral vasoconstriction
  - Dexamethasone (12–16 mg daily) to reduce vasogenic oedema
  - Neurosurgical drainage of CSF, decompression, or decompressive craniectomy

Obstructive hydrocephalus

- Due to blockage of the CSF pathway and the causes include:
  - Congenital malformation: Aqueduct stenosis, Dandy-Walker syndrome
  - Chronic meningitis: tuberculosis, cryptococcus, malignant infiltration
  - Mass lesion: haematoma, abscess, intrinsic or extrinsic tumour
  - Others: SAH, aneurysm, colloid cyst, spina bifida

- CT or MRI brain features: dilated ventricles with rounded horns, periventricular lucencies, flattened subarachnoid space with effacement of cerebral sulci; possibly the causative lesion
- Neurosurgical treatment is shunting (e.g., external drainage or ventriculoperitoneal shunt). Possible complications are over-shunting (may lead to low ICP or subdural haematoma), infection (resulting in meningitis and ventriculitis), and blockage.

Normal pressure hydrocephalus (communicating hydrocephalus)

This term refers to chronic hydrocephalus with intermittently raised CSF pressure, typically presenting with a triad of:
- Gait dyspraxia with initiation difficulty and postural instability
- Mental impairment usually affecting frontal lobe functions, e.g., forgetfulness (usually a retrieval deficit rather than defective encoding), inertia, bradyphrenia, apathy, inattention, impaired judgement, and delayed recall
- Urinary incontinence with urgency

MRI brain shows ventricular enlargement out of proportion to peripheral sulcal enlargement $\pm$ periventricular radiolucency (increased T_2 weighted or FLAIR signal due to transependymal fluid shift). CSF flow study may aid diagnosis in difficult cases.

Management

- External lumbar drainage of CSF (40–100 ml) to test for clinical improvement, e.g., notably gait performance in 72 hours.
- For doubtful cases, slow continuous CSF drainage for 3–5 days $\pm$ ICP monitoring to document intermittently raised CSF pressure may improve the test sensitivity.
- Permanent ventriculo-peritoneal shunting for definite cases
- Complications of shunting include orthostatic headache, subdural haematoma or hygroma, which may be prevented by adjustment of shunt-valve pressure. Shunt infection is rare, but removal or reinsertion is sometimes required.

Idiopathic intracranial hypertension (benign intracranial hypertension, pseudotumour cerebri)

It is due to a combination of increased CSF outflow resistance and decreased CSF absorption. It is more common in females and tends to occur in obese women of childbearing age. ICP is raised (> 25 cm water at LP) without any space-occupying lesion or obstruction of the CSF pathways. On CT or MRI brain, the ventricles are small or normal, and the sella may be enlarged and filled with CSF (empty-sella syndrome). Patients present with features of raised ICP, but no cause is found in most cases. CSF findings are normal. Important differential diagnoses are cerebral venous thrombosis, chronic meningitis, and choroid plexus papilloma. A number of systemic diseases (e.g., Behçet's disease, SLE) and drugs (e.g., oestrogen, phenytoin, steroid therapy or withdrawal) are known to be associated with this condition.

Treatment

Although rarely life-threatening, raised ICP may damage the optic nerves and cause permanent visual loss. Constriction of peripheral visual field and enlargement of blind spot due to papilledema are characteristic. Treatment includes repeated LP to remove CSF, a short course of oral prednisolone or acetazolamide, and dieting to lose weight. Surgical intervention (e.g., lumboperitoneal shunt, optic nerve fenestration) may be required if vision is threatened. Spontaneous relapses and remissions are common.

Acute mountain sickness

It is associated with subacute cerebral hypoxia, and presents with headache, nausea, insomnia, and impaired concentration. It begins within several days of ascending a height above 3,000 metres. Pulmonary and cerebral oedema and coma with possible fatality may ensue if left untreated, or if the patient does not descend quickly. Treatment is by corticosteroids and oxygen. Acetazolamide may prevent this condition.

Intracranial hypotension

Post-LP headache

It occurs in 5% of patients and is caused by leakage of CSF at the needle site. The use of a smaller needle, e.g., 22G or below and replacement of stylet, helps to minimize the incidence. The typical symptom is orthostatic headache, accompanied by stiff neck, nausea, vomiting, tinnitus or altered hearing. It is promptly relieved by lying down. Traction on cranial nerve root may result in abducens paralysis and hence horizontal diplopia. MRI with gadolinium may show dural enhancement or a pocket of CSF at site of leakage. Dural blood (autologous) patch is effective if headache persists despite conservative management.

Spontaneous intracranial hypotension

The typical symptom is intense headache in the erect position, which is relieved upon lying down. This results from leakage of CSF. The cause may not be apparent in some cases and presumably an arachnoid tear (usually at the thoracic or lumbar segment) has occurred. In other cases, it may follow excessive straining, accidental dural puncture in epidural anaesthesia, spine fracture, and fracture of cribriform plate.

Low or negative opening pressure at LP, CSF pleocytosis, and modest elevation of protein level are present. MRI brain typically shows diffuse dural enhancement due to compensatory increase in intracranial blood volume. CSF flow study on MRI brain and MRI spine with intrathecal contrast may help to identify the site of leakage. Most patients recover after conservative treatment, e.g., analgesics, bed rest, and IV saline replacement. Multiple dural blood patches to the leakage site may be required in resistant case. Surgical repair of the dura is required in appropriate cases.

6 Cerebrovascular Disease

Cerebrovascular disease or stroke ranks first in frequency and importance among all adult neurological diseases. It encompasses any abnormality of the brain due to various pathological changes in the cerebral vessels, including vessel wall lesion, thrombotic or embolic occlusion of the lumen, vascular rupture, altered vascular permeability, vascular malformation, hypercoagulability, bleeding tendency, and hyperviscosity. The results are stroke, transient ischaemic attack (TIA), cerebral venous thrombosis, and vascular dementia (see Chapter 11).

Stroke is a syndrome of rapidly developing clinical symptoms and signs of focal or global disturbance of cerebral functions due to non-traumatic vascular causes, with symptoms lasting more than 24 hours or rapidly leading to death. As a cerebrovascular insult, stroke is popularly yet inappropriately called a cerebrovascular accident (CVA). In TIA, the clinical features of stroke completely resolve within 24 hours without evidence of brain infarction on neuroimaging. TIA is also known as mini-stroke, and most TIAs last less than 1 hour. Following repeated strokes, vascular dementia may become evident.

Types and subtypes of stroke

Stroke is not a homogeneous disease. Major types of stroke (Figure 6.1) are ischaemic stroke (ISS; in about 70% of patients), intracerebral haemorrhage (ICH; in about 25% of patients), and subarachnoid haemorrhage (SAH; in about 5% of patients). Spinal cord stroke and cerebral venous thrombosis are rare.

Subtypes of ISS include cortical, subcortical, posterior circulation, and lacunar infarction. The common pathogenic mechanisms

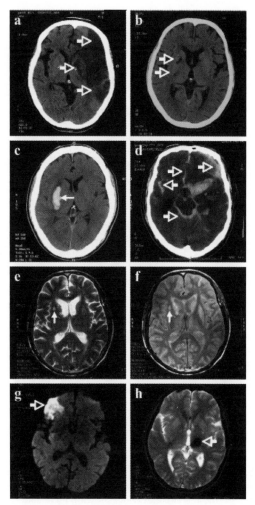

Figure 6.1 CT brain with the arrow(s) pointing at (a) an extensive left middle cerebral artery infarction, (b) two lacunar infarctions at right basal ganglia, (c) supratentorial ICH and (d) extensive SAH plus obstructive hydrocephalus. MRI brain with the arrow pointing at a tiny lacunar infarction at right basal ganglia on (e) T_2 weighted or (f) proton density image, (g) an acute infarction over the anterior part of right middle cerebral artery territory, and (h) blooming of old blood products on gradient-echo T2* image.

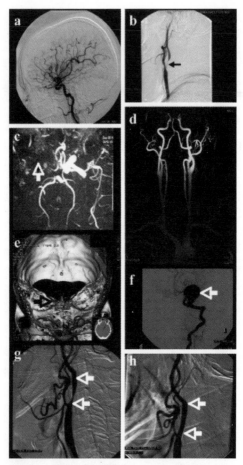

Figure 6.2 Digital subtraction angiography showing (a) normal intracranial vasculature and (b) severe stenosis of the left ICA (arrow). MRA
of the brain around the circle of Willis showing (c) absent right middle
cerebral artery (arrow) due to occlusion of the right ICA. Gadolinium-
enhanced MRA of the neck showing (d) normal appearance of the
major arteries arising from the aortic arch to the brain. CTA of the
brain around the circle of Willis showing (e) absent right middle cerebral artery (arrow) in relation to the skull base. Digital subtraction
angiography showing (f) a giant tip of basilar aneurysm (arrow), and
deployment of stent (arrows) to the left ICA (g) before and (h) after
post-stenting dilatation.

of ISS include atherothrombosis, artery-to-artery embolism, cardi-oembolism, and small vessel disease (Table 6.1). Atherothrombosis can result in massive infarction involving the entire territory of the ICA, middle cerebral artery or basilar artery. Artery-to-artery embolism and cardioembolism tend to produce smaller cortical infarction. Small vessel disease results in lacunar infarction and leukoaraiosis (Binswanger's disease).

ICH can be classified into supratentorial or infratentorial ICH. The leading causes of ICH are hypertensive micro-aneurysm, aneurysm, arteriovenous malformation (AVM) and bleeding ten-dency (Table 6.2).

SAH is commonly caused by ruptured aneurysm or AVM.

Table 6.1   Pathogenic mechanisms of ISS

Mechanism	Causes/risk factors
Atherothrombosis	Hypertension
	Diabetes mellitus
	Hypercholesterolaemia
	Cigarette smoking
	Coronary artery disease
	Central obesity
	Physical inactivity
	Male gender
	Family history
Artery-to-artery embolism	As above
Cardioembolism	Valvular heart disease
	Non-valvular AF
	Infective endocarditis
	Acute myocardial infarction
	Left ventricular aneurysm
	Cardiomyopathy
	Left atrial myxoma
	Sick sinus syndrome
	Paradoxical embolism via septal defects
Small vessel disease	Hypertension
	Advancing age
	Diabetes mellitus
	Cerebral amyloid angiopathy

Table 6.1 (continued)

Haemodynamic failure	Cardiac failure
	Hypovolaemia
	Hypotension
	Vasoconstriction
Hypercoagulability	Pregnancy
	Peripartum and postpartum states
	Use of oral contraceptives
	Anti-phospholipid antibody syndrome
	Protein C or S deficiency
	Polycythaemia or thrombocytosis
	Nephrotic syndrome
	Dysproteinaemia
	Anti-thrombin III deficiency
	Increased factor VIII
Other arterial diseases	Arterial dissection
	Moyamoya disease
	Takayasu disease
	Cranial arteritis
	Vasculitis
	Post-irradiation vasculopathy

Table 6.2 Location of intracranial haemorrhage by causes

Cause	Locations
Hypertension	Basal ganglia, lobar, pons, cerebellum
Bleeding tendency (heparin, warfarin, NOACs, leukaemia, haemophilia, thrombocytopaenia)	Lobar, cerebellar, subarachnoid, multifocal
Cerebral amyloid angiopathy	Lobar, subarachnoid, recurrent or multifocal
Vascular abnormality (aneurysm, AVM, Moyamoya disease)	Subarachnoid, ventricular, parenchymal
Illicit drugs (cocaine, amphetamine)	Subarachnoid, intracerebral
Brain tumours	Multifocal, junction between grey and white matter site of primary tumour

In general, small vessel disease occurs more often in Orientals. Lacunar stroke can manifest as pure motor hemiparesis, pure sensory stroke, sensorimotor stroke, clumsy hand dysarthria syndrome, ataxic hemiparesis or other specific patterns. Pathologically, lacunar stroke is most commonly due to lacunar infarct but is rarely due to a small ICH. Occlusion of small penetrating arteries due to lipohyalinosis and fibrinoid degeneration produces small (1–15 mm in diameter), irregular infarcts in the striatum, thalamus, internal capsule, corona radiata, and brainstem. The major risk factors are hypertension (in over 70% of patients) and DM.

Cortical infarct is characterized by the presence of cortical signs (e.g., dysphasia, dyspraxia, homonymous hemianopia, conjugate gaze palsy).

Mortality and morbidity

Globally, stroke is the second leading cause of death and a major cause of morbidity and disability. However, mortality and morbidity vary with different stroke types and subtypes. In SAH, half of the patients die within the first month, and over half of the survivors have severe morbidity. About 40% of patients with ICH die at one month and 50% at one year. Mortality is relatively high in cortical infarct (about 20% at one month and 35% at one year) but low in lacunar infarct (less than 1% at one month and 2% at one year). Morbidity is worse in survivors of cortical infarct than ICH, whereas survivors of lacunar infarct have milder disability and are ambulatory and independent in activities of daily living (ADL; see Chapter 19). The modified Rankin Scale (mRS) is the most widely used clinical outcome measure for disability after stroke in clinical trials (Table 6.3).

Table 6.3   Modified Rankin Scale (mRS)

Best description of disability	Score
No symptom at all	0
No significant disability despite symptoms: able to carry out all usual duties and activities	1
Slight disability: unable to carry out all previous activities but able to look after own affairs without assistance	2
Moderate disability: requiring some help but able to walk without assistance	3
Moderately severe disability: unable to walk without assistance and unable to attend to body needs without assistance	4
Severe disability: bedridden, incontinent and requiring constant nursing care and attention	5
Death	6

Clinical features

The onset of stroke is sudden in most cases. Symptoms and signs of stroke reflect the location and extent of damage, hence the importance of a working knowledge of the anatomy of cerebral arteries. Neurological deficits should be documented in a systemic manner using the National Institutes of Health Stroke Scale (NIHSS; Table 6.4).

In carotid territory stroke, the clinical features include hemiparesis, hemifacial weakness, hemisensory loss, dysphasia (dominant hemisphere), visuospatial disorientation (non-dominant hemisphere), dysarthria, deviation of head and eyes towards the lesion side, and dysphagia.

In vertebrobasilar stroke, the clinical features include cortical blindness, homonymous visual field defects, diplopia, nystagmus, vertigo, Horner's syndrome, dysarthria, dysphagia, cranial nerve deficits, hemiparesis, tetraparesis, unilateral sensory loss, bilateral sensory loss, and ataxia.

In SAH, the cardinal feature is severe headache of sudden onset. Neck stiffness takes hours to develop, and consciousness is impaired in severe cases. Subhyaloid haemorrhagic (Figure 3.4h) may be present.

Table 6.4   National Institutes of Health Stroke Scale (NIHSS)

Item	Description	Score
Level of consciousness	Alert, keenly responsive	0
	Drowsy, arousable by minor stimulation	1
	Unresponsive or only reflex response	2
Level of consciousness by questions (age, month)	Both correct	0
	One correct	1
	Both incorrect	2
Level of consciousness by commands (close eye, make a fist)	Both correct	0
	One correct	1
	Both incorrect	2
Best gaze (horizontal)	Full range of eye movements	0
	Partial gaze palsy or isolated nerve palsy	1
	Forced deviation or total gaze paresis	2
Best visual field	Normal	0
	Asymmetry or partial hemianopia	1
	Complete hemianopia	2
	Bilateral hemianopia or coma	3
Facial weakness	None or sedated	0
	Minor or loss of nasolabial fold	1
	Partial or lower face	2
	Complete or coma	3
Best motor left arm	Held at 90 degrees for 10s	0
	Drift within 10s	1
	Fall within 10s but some effort against gravity	2
	Slight movements with no effort against gravity	3
	No movement	4
Best motor right arm	Held at 90 degrees for 10s	0
	Drift within 10s	1
	Fall within 10s but some effort against gravity	2
	Slight movements with no effort against gravity	3
	No movement	4

Table 6.4   (continued)

Item	Description	Score
Best motor left leg	Held at 30 degrees for 5s	0
	Drift within 5s	1
	Fall within 5s but some effort against gravity	2
	Slight movements with no effort against gravity	3
	No movement	4
Best motor right leg	Held at 30 degrees for 5s	0
	Drift within 5s	1
	Fall within 5s but some effort against gravity	2
	Slight movements with no effort against gravity	3
	No movement	4
Best language	Normal	0
	Mild to moderate aphasia	1
	Severe aphasia	2
	Mute or global aphasia or coma	3
Articulation	Normal	0
	Mild to moderate dysarthria	1
	Severe dysarthria or mute	2
Limb ataxia (finger-to-nose, heel-shin test)	Absent or cannot be examined	0
	Ataxia in one limb	1
	Ataxia in two or more limbs	2
Pinprick sensation	Normal	0
	Mild to moderate loss	1
	Severe or total loss or coma	2
Neglect	No neglect	0
	Visual or tactile inattention	1
	Visual and tactile inattention or coma	2

Differential diagnosis of stroke

- Intracranial tumour
- Epidural or chronic subdural haematoma
- Encephalitis
- Multiple sclerosis

- Seizure, e.g., Todd's paralysis
- Hypoglycaemia
- Drug intoxication
- Brain abscess
- Craniocervical trauma
- Complicated migraine
- Functional disorders

Complications

Many cerebral or systemic complications can occur.
- Cerebral complications
  - Cerebral oedema
  - Raised ICP, hydrocephalus
  - Herniation
  - Haemorrhagic transformation of cerebral infarction
  - Seizures
- Systemic complications of stroke
  - Pneumonia: hypostatic, aspiration
  - Deep vein thrombosis ± pulmonary embolism
  - Pressure sores
  - Urinary tract infection
  - Cardiovascular disturbance
  - Fluid and electrolytes disturbance
  - Contractures, frozen shoulder
  - Anxiety, depression

Approach to stroke

Stroke is a neurological emergency, hence the term 'brain attack'. Management of stroke begins with an accurate diagnosis and classification of stroke types from history, physical examination and investigations. The aims of initial evaluation are to assess vital signs, confirm the diagnosis, differentiate ischaemic from haemorrhagic strokes, provide clues on the most likely aetiology, and screen for early complications.

Investigations

- Neuroimaging is mandatory in stroke therapy. Plain CT brain effectively excludes intracranial haemorrhage (Figure 6.1).
- MRI (Figure 6.1) is superior to CT in revealing small infarcts or lesions in the posterior fossa, but it requires a longer scanning time. It is contraindicated in patients with claustrophobia, pacemaker (most older models) or metallic implants. Patients implanted with new MRI-conditional pacemakers can safely undergo MRI using 1.5T machines. MRI brain, MRA brain and neck (stroke package) are usually arranged.
- Cerebral angiography (conventional or digital subtraction; MRA, CTA, Figure 6.2), transcranial Doppler, and duplex ultrasound examination of the cervical arteries can detect arterial diseases such as atherosclerosis and dissection.
- In SAH, CT shows blood in the subarachnoid space or ventricles in 95% of patients within 24 hours of onset. LP should be done in CT negative cases if there is a strong suspicion of SAH. The CSF may be bloodstained or xanthochromic, depending on the time elapsed since the ictus.
- ECG
- CXR for suspected pneumonia and/or heart failure
- Trans-thoracic and trans-esophageal echocardiography and Holter monitoring for patients with suspected cardiogenic embolism
- CBC, ESR, LFT, RFT, PT, APTT, fasting blood glucose and lipids
- Special haematological and serological tests for patients with suspected hypercoagulability, antiphospholipid antibody syndrome, and vasculitis

General management

These measures stabilize the patient's conditions and prevent complications, and are of equal importance as specific treatments in improving outcome.

1. Manage in an Acute Stroke Unit (ASU) if available. ASU is an acute neurological ward providing specialist services for patients suspected to have a new stroke.
2. Check eligibility for intravenous thrombolysis.
3. Closely monitor neurological and vital signs.
4. Maintain adequate tissue oxygenation. Avoid hypoxia via prevention of airway obstruction, hypoventilation, aspiration pneumonia, and atelectasis. Treat hypoxia with oxygen, endotracheal intubation, and/or assisted ventilation. Hyperbaric oxygen has no proven value in improving stroke outcome.
5. Commence osmotherapy and hyperventilation for raised ICP. Do not use corticosteroids.
6. Use AEDs for recurrent seizures; seizures complicate <10% of patients with ISS (especially with haemorrhagic transformation); early onset (within 1 week) seizures occur in up to 16% of patients with ICH (especially with lobar ICH); seizures are relatively common (up to 26%) after SAH; short-term use of prophylactic AEDs may be considered in the immediate post-haemorrhagic period.
7. Elevated BP is commonly observed at the early stage of stroke, but rapid or drastic reduction is not required for mildly to moderately raised BP. Lowering BP in acute stroke may decrease cerebral perfusion in patients with critical stenosis of major arteries.
8. Hyperthermia aggravates brain damage. Treat infection vigorously and lower the core temperature.
9. Risk of deep vein thrombosis and pulmonary embolism can be reduced by early mobilization, external compression devices, and subcutaneous heparin or low-molecular-weight heparin (LMWH).
10. Avoid electrolyte imbalance, hypovolaemia, and fluid overload.
11. Use tube-feeding for patients with impaired gag reflex, depressed consciousness or dysphagia. Maintain euglycaemia.
12. Avoid over-distension of the bladder and urinary tract infection. Use urinary catheter when needed.
13. Avoid constipation, faecal impaction or soiling by providing high-fibre diet and stool softener.

14. Arrange frequent turning (e.g., every 2 hours), air mattress, physiotherapy, and occupational therapy to prevent pressure sores and contractures.
15. Consult speech therapists for dysphagia, dysarthria, or dysphasia.
16. Look out for and treat depression, insomnia or other psychiatric complications.

Acute therapy for ISS

Normal neuronal functions require continuous supply of oxygen and glucose coupled with efficient removal of metabolic waste. A moderate mismatch between energy supply and metabolic demand causes reversible dysfunction (the ischaemic penumbra), whereas a severe mismatch results in rapid neuronal death (the ischaemic core). This unstable ischaemic penumbra provides an opportunity for acute intervention within the therapeutic time window. Acute thrombolysis offers proven benefit, but results of clinical trials on neuroprotectants have so far been disappointing.

Acute thrombolysis

IV recombinant tissue plasminogen activator (tPA) at 0.9 mg/kg (10% as bolus and 90% infusion over 1 hour) commenced within 3 hours of onset increases the proportion of patients with minimal or no disability by 13%. Despite an increased risk of symptomatic ICH, mortality is slightly reduced in the tPA patients. Other complications include major systemic haemorrhage and angioedema. Patient selection is crucial, and the inclusion and exclusion criteria (Table 6.5) should be adhered to. Treatment after 3 hours but within 4.5 hours of onset is also effective, and the proportion of patients with very good outcome can be increased by 7%. However, additional exclusion criteria should be observed.

Large artery occlusion responds poorly to IV thrombolysis with a low recanalization rate between 15% and 30%; endovascular treatment with mechanical thrombectomy devices can achieve a high recanalization rate between 60% and 85%. Approved devices include a coil retriever, an aspiration system, and stent retrievers. Endovascular treatment requires specially trained neuro-interventionalists, dedicated angiography room with experienced staffs, appropriate anaesthesia or sedation and intensive care support. Treatment time window can be up to 8 hours of onset of large artery occlusion in the anterior circulation. Endovascular treatment should not preclude eligible patients from receiving IV thrombolysis. It is the treatment of choice in certain cases when IV thrombolysis is contraindicated. It is considered a salvage therapy in patients with acute basilar artery occlusion. Complications include device fracture, vessel dissection, perforation and occlusion, intracranial haemorrhage and non-target artery embolization.

The narrow treatment time window for intravenous thrombolysis or endovascular treatment will exclude the great majority of stroke patients. Effective public education may shorten the delay in hospital presentation of stroke patients.

Table 6.5   Inclusion and exclusion criteria for IV tPA

Inclusion criteria	Exclusion criteria
Acute ISS in any territory with measurable deficit	History of intracranial haemorrhage
	Intracranial neoplasm, AVM or aneurysm
Witnessed onset time or time last seen well < 3 hours	Suspected SAH
	Significant head trauma or stroke in previous 3 months
Age 18 or older	GI or urinary bleeding within 3 weeks
Potential risks and benefits discussed with AND understood by patient and/or family members	Intracranial, intraspinal or major surgery in previous 2 weeks
	Arterial puncture at noncompressible site in previous 1 week
	Platelet < 100,000 per cu mm
	Use of heparin within 48 hours with prolonged APTT
	INR > 1.7 or PT > 15s
	Use of NOACs

Anticoagulation

Evidence from clinical trials does not support the general use of anticoagulation in acute ISS. Possible indications for early anticoagulation in ISS include progressing stroke, high risk of cardiogenic embolism, prevention of DVT and pulmonary embolism, cerebral venous thrombosis and hypercoagulability. The potential benefit has to be balanced against the increased risk of haemorrhagic transformation of infarction, as spontaneous haemorrhagic transformation is not uncommon and usually occurs within 2–4 days of onset. Other contraindications of anticoagulation should be observed.

Antiplatelet therapy in acute stage

Early use of low-dose aspirin (160–300 mg daily) within 48 hours of onset is a cost-effective treatment for patients with ISS: a reduction of 11 recurrent ISS or deaths but with two extra cases of haemorrhagic transformation for each thousand patients treated.

Role of neurosurgery

- Monitor ICP.
- Control markedly raised ICP when medical therapy fails.
- Consider surgical decompression of large non-dominant hemispheric infarct in young patients, e.g., infarctectomy, decompressive craniectomy.
- Cerebellar infarction carries a significant risk of direct brainstem compression and obstructive hydrocephalus. Consider drainage of hydrocephalus, infarctectomy or posterior fossa decompression.

Management of ICH

Control of BP

This is crucial, as uncontrolled hypertension predisposes to continual bleeding. Consider the patient's pre-stroke BP, and avoid any precipitous drop. Consider ß-blockers, calcium antagonists or angiotensin converting enzyme inhibitors.

Patients with bleeding diatheses

The underlying disorders (Table 6.2) should be treated. Stop and reverse any anticoagulation promptly and completely by appropriate measures, e.g., protamine sulphate, fresh frozen plasma, parenteral vitamin K_1, recombinant activated factor VII. Aim at normal PT, APTT and adequate platelet counts. Preservation of brain function takes priority over any indication of anticoagulation. When the neurological condition becomes stable for 7–10 days, cautiously resume anticoagulation if indicated, e.g., prosthetic heart valve.

Control of raised ICP

Raised ICP may depress consciousness and respiration and cause death. Repeat CT brain in case of deterioration. Medical therapy of raised ICP includes control of BP, fluid restriction, osmotic agents (mannitol), and mechanical ventilation to keep $PaCO_2$ at 25 mmHg. Consider ICP monitoring and surgical decompression.

Neurosurgical referral

In general, evacuation of large deep cerebral haematoma improves survival but not quality of life. Adopt conservative treatment for brainstem haemorrhage. However, prompt neurosurgical treatment reduces mortality and morbidity in the following conditions:
- Acute hydrocephalus due to obstruction of CSF flow: ventricular drainage (also permit ICP monitoring) or ventriculoperitoneal shunting
- Cerebellar haematoma: clot evacuation or ventricular drainage
- Large superficial or lobar haematoma with marked deficits
- Intraventricular haemorrhage with hydrocephalus: ventricular drainage and thrombolysis of intraventricular clots

Management of SAH

- SAH is an emergency and neurosurgeons should be consulted urgently.

- Prevent and treat complications; deterioration is often due to one or more complications.
  - Rebleeding: incidence peaks in the first 24 hours of aneurysmal SAH and markedly decreases after the first 2 weeks. Rebleeding is preventable by clipping the aneurysm. Antifibrinolytic drugs (e.g., tranexamic acid, aminocaproic acid) reduce the risk of rebleeding but may provoke vasospasm.
  - Vasospasm and cerebral ischaemia: incidence is highest between 4 and 14 days of aneurysmal SAH. Calcium antagonist (e.g., nimodipine 60 mg orally every 4 hours for 21 days), triple-H therapy (for hypertension, hypervolaemia, and haemodilution; safe after clipping of the aneurysm), transluminal angioplasty, and intra-arterial papaverine are treatment options.
  - Acute hydrocephalus
  - Cerebral oedema
  - Seizure
  - Syndrome of inappropriate antidiuretic hormone (SIADH)
  - Cardiac arrhythmia
  - Other systemic complications, e.g., pneumonia, urinary tract infection, DVT
- Definitive treatment of the underlying lesion to prevent recurrence
  - Arrange urgent cerebral angiography
  - Obliterate aneurysm: neurosurgery or endovascular procedures

Less common entities

Dissection of cerebral arteries

Cervicocephalic arterial dissection is not uncommon and should be considered in young patients with stroke. It may occur spontaneously or follow penetrating or blunt trauma. Fibromuscular dysplasia is an underlying cause in some patients. Antecedent events include neck manipulation, competitive sports, and yoga. The extracranial ICA is more commonly affected than the vertebral artery; intracranial arterial dissection is uncommon. Typical symptoms include headache or neck pain, cerebral ischaemic symptoms (TIA, stroke), and Horner's syndrome. Cerebral angiography, Doppler sonography, and MRI plus MRA are useful diagnostic tests. Treatment remains controversial. Anticoagulation for 3–6 months is often used in patients with cerebral ischaemic symptoms in the absence of large infarction, or intracranial dissection or haemorrhage. Good clinical and angiographic recovery usually occurs in patients with spontaneous dissection.

AVM

This is the vascular anomaly connecting the arteries and veins and therefore bypassing the capillary. AVMs are usually congenital and asymptomatic. Symptoms are related to the location, expansion, and bleeding (e.g., ICH or SAH). Common symptoms are headache, epilepsy, acute focal neurologic deficits, and progressive neurologic deficits. Young children with large AVMs can present with heart failure, macrocephaly, and prominent scalp veins. Plain CT may reveal recent haemorrhage in the form of ICH, SAH, or multiple foci of calcification along vascular channels. CT with contrast shows abnormal enhancement. MRI can reveal a tangle of vascular channels as flow voids. CTA or MRA may be adequate for initial or follow-up evaluation of an AVM. However, digital subtraction angiography remains the gold standard for delineation and characterization of an AVM and provides information on the feeders, venous drainage, associated aneurysms, and venous stenosis. Treatment depends on the presenting symptoms, location and size of the AVM, and the risk of bleeding. Surgical resection can be curative. Radiosurgery with gamma knife or X-knife can induce complete obliteration of small or deep AVMs several years after treatment. Endovascular embolization of the feeders with glue is an adjunctive treatment.

Moyamoya disease

This is a progressive occlusive disease of the cerebral vasculature with particular involvement of the circle of Willis and its feeding arteries. The aetiology is unknown. It is much more common in Asians. Most patients present in the first decades, and others in the third and fourth decades. Children can be asymptomatic or have TIA or ISS, whereas adults usually present with ICH or SAH. Cognitive decline occurs after recurrent strokes. Cerebral angiography is diagnostic, and MRA or CTA may provide similar information (Figure 6.2). Characteristic findings are bilateral stenosis or occlusion at the terminal segment of the ICA or the proximal segment of the anterior, middle or posterior cerebral arteries with nearby abnormal vascular collateral networks appearing as a 'puff of smoke' (*moyamoya* in Japanese). Treatment is directed primarily at complications. Preventive strategy depends on the angiographic findings, type and severity of stroke, and risk-to-benefit analysis of antithrombotic therapy. Neurosurgical revascularization procedures have been advocated.

Cerebral venous thrombosis

This is an uncommon but potentially serious type of stroke. Thrombosis may affect the cortical or deep cerebral veins or the straight, sagittal, transverse, sigmoid and/or cavernous sinus. Generalized or local infection is the primary aetiology in less developed countries. Non-infectious causes include hypercoagulable states, haematological disorders, chronic inflammatory diseases, systemic or local neoplastic conditions, dehydration or flow disorders, drug or hormonal use, pregnancy, and postoperative state. Clinical features may be non-specific, but features of raised ICP, seizures and focal signs are common. MRI and MR venography are diagnostic. Treatment consists of anticoagulation, AED, control of raised ICP, supportive measures, and management of the underlying cause.

Rehabilitation (see Chapter 19)

This is an essential aspect of stroke management as one-third of patients would have at least moderate impairment and disability.

Prevention of stroke

Prevention is the best strategy to reduce the burden of stroke. Primary prevention is prevention of stroke in people with no history of cerebrovascular symptoms, and secondary prevention applies to patients who have had a stroke or TIA. Epidemiological and cohort studies have revealed many modifiable risk factors for stroke (Table 6.6). Risk factor screening not only identifies people at risk of stroke but also encourages a healthy lifestyle in the general population.

Hypertension

Hypertension is the major predisposing factor for atherosclerosis in large and medium-sized arteries, arteriolosclerosis in small penetrating arteries, cardiac diseases of ischaemic and hypertensive types, and hypertensive micro-aneurysms. These pathological processes may cause stroke through atherothrombosis, embolism, occlusion of small vessels or arterial rupture.

Table 6.6   Risk factors for stroke

Category	Action to prevent stroke
Modifiable factors	
• Previous stroke or TIA	Consider long-term antiplatelet agents or anticoagulation
• Hypertension	Screen for hypertension; keep systolic and diastolic BP below 140 and 85 mmHg, respectively
• Cardiac diseases	Screen for cardiac diseases
• Atrial fibrillation	Check ECG and echocardiography; consider long-term anticoagulation or antiplatelet agents

Table 6.6   (continued)

Category	Action to prevent stroke
• DM	Screen for undiagnosed DM; aim at strict glycaemic control
• ICA stenosis	Check carotid ultrasound, MRA or CTA; consider carotid endarterectomy or percutaneous carotid angioplasty with stenting
• Cigarette smoking	Quit smoking; consider nicotine gum or pad
• Alcohol abuse	Reduce consumption
• Hypercholesterolaemia	Screen for dyslipoproteinaemia; consider dietary control and 'statins'
• Obesity	Reduce weight
• Lack of exercise	Regular exercise
• Haematological abnormalities, coagulopathies	Screen for and treat the underlying disorders

Non-modifiable risk factors
- Advancing age
- Male sex
- Family history
- Race

Cardiogenic causes

About a quarter of all ISSs are embolic in nature (Table 6.7). The mere presence of a potential cardioembolic source in a stroke patient may be coincidental, and other possible causes of stroke should be considered. Different cardiac conditions carry different risks of stroke (Table 6.8). Long-term antithrombotic therapy reduces the risk of embolic stroke but at the expense of an increased risk of systemic and cerebral haemorrhage.

Table 6.7   Features suggesting embolic stroke

Clinical features	Presence of a cardioembolic source Non-progressive onset Non-lacunar stroke Cortical deficit: hemianopia, aphasia or ideomotor apraxia Lack of vascular risk factors No other cause of stroke
Topographical features	Posterior division of the middle cerebral artery Anterior cerebral artery Cerebellar arteries Multiple territories
Radiological features	Superficial cortical location in the above territories Multifocal infarcts Haemorrhagic transformation on CT Embolic occlusion without atherosclerosis or normal findings in angiography

Table 6.8   Causes and management of cardioembolic stroke

Type	Example	Management
Valvular heart disease	Rheumatic heart disease, prosthetic valves	Anticoagulation
	Infective endocarditis	Antibiotics
	Calcific aortic stenosis, mitral valve prolapse	?Aspirin
	Mitral annulus calcification	Anticoagulation, surgery
	Non-bacterial thrombotic endocarditis	Aspirin, ?anticoagulation
	Inflammatory valvulitis	Treat underlying cause
Coronary heart disease	Acute myocardial infarction	Anticoagulation
	Left ventricular aneurysm or dyskinesia	?Anticoagulation
Arrhythmia	Atrial fibrillation	Anticoagulation, aspirin
	Sick sinus syndrome	Pacemaker, anticoagulation
Cardiomyopathy	Dilating cardiomyopathy	Anticoagulation
	Hypertrophic cardiomyopathy	ß-blocker, surgery
Tumour	Primary atrial myxoma	Surgery
Paradoxical emboli	Atrial septal defects	Surgery, ?anticoagulation
	Patent foramen ovale	?Anticoagulation
	Ventricular septal defects	Surgery, ?anticoagulation

? = controversial

About 1% of the general population, 6% of people aged above 65 years and 10% of those over 75 years have atrial fibrillation; non-valvular AF is the most common cause. Systemic embolization of stasis-induced left atrial thrombi may produce ISS. Patients with non-valvular AF have an increased risk of stroke, and the actual risk can be estimated using clinical prediction schemes such as CHA_2DS_2-VASc score (Tables 6.9 and 6.10). Long-term use of warfarin (with INR 2–3) reduces the risk by about 60%, and use of low dose aspirin (100–300 mg daily) reduces the risk by about 20%. Anticoagulation is recommended to males with CHA_2DS_2-VASc score ≥ 1 and females with score ≥ 2.

Table 6.9 CHA_2DS_2-VASc score for patients with non-valvular AF

Acronym	Condition	Points
C	Congestive heart failure	1
H	Hypertension	1
A2	Age ≥ 75 years	2
D	Diabetes mellitus	1
S2	Prior stroke or TIA or thromboembolism	2
V	Vascular disease (e.g., peripheral, coronary)	1
A	Age 65–74 years	1
Sc	Sex category (i.e., female gender)	1

Table 6.10   Annual stroke risk according to CHA_2DS_2-VASc score

Score	Annual stroke risk %
0	0
1	1.3
2	2.2
3	3.2
4	4.0
5	6.7
6	9.8
7	9.6
8	12.5
9	15.2

Patients with AF and rheumatic heart disease need long-term anticoagulation. Anticoagulation carries 1–2% annual risk of severe bleeding, including 0.3% annual incidence of ICH.

New oral anticoagulants (NOACs) are available as the alternative to warfarin for the prevention and treatment of thrombosis. NOACs target either thrombin (dabigatran etexilate) or factor Xa (rivaroxaban and apixaban). Advantages of NOACs include rapid onset/offset of action, few drug/food interactions, and predictable pharmacokinetics; regular coagulation monitoring is not useful or unnecessary. Efficacy and safety are not inferior to warfarin for stroke prevention in non-valvular AF and for treatment and secondary prevention of venous thromboembolism. For initial treatment of venous thromboembolism and thromboprophylaxis in patients undergoing hip or knee arthroplasty, their efficacy is comparable to LMWH. Disadvantages include a lack of laboratory monitoring for compliance, uncertainty about dosing in selected patient populations (e.g., renal impairment, extremes of body weight), and high drug cost. Specific antidote is available for dabigatran.

DM

DM is associated with both atherothrombotic stroke and stroke due to small vessel disease. Since undiagnosed DM is common in the elderly population, screening is important.

Chronic smoking

Chronic smoking increases the risk of stroke of all types, and the risk is proportional to the number of cigarettes consumed per day. The risk decreases promptly towards the level of non-smokers within five years of quitting.

Alcohol

Alcohol intake of low to moderate level (1–2 drinks per day) reduces the risk for ISS and coronary heart disease, whereas heavy drinking increases the risk for ischaemic and haemorrhagic strokes.

Dyslipoproteinaemia

Dyslipoproteinaemia is due to a high level of total or low-density lipoprotein cholesterol, a reduced level of high-density lipoprotein cholesterol, an increased ratio of low- to high-density lipoprotein cholesterols, or a combination of these. Statins (HMG-CoA reductase inhibitors) reduces the risk of fatal and non-fatal strokes as well as retards the progression of carotid atherosclerosis.

Antithrombotic therapy

Anticoagulation

Long-term anticoagulation is indicated in patients with a high risk of embolic events (Tables 6.7 and 6.8).

Antiplatelet agents

Use of aspirin for primary prevention of stroke among healthy subjects is controversial. Low-dose aspirin reduces the risk of myocardial infarction, but there is a small increase in the incidence of ICH.

For secondary prevention, aspirin reduces vascular mortality by about 15% and non-fatal vascular events (stroke and myocardial infarction) by about 30%. A daily dosage of 75–300 mg is as effective as 1.3 gm daily. A combination of low-dose aspirin and a slow-release form of dipyridamole is better than aspirin alone. Clopidogrel (75 mg daily) is also more effective than aspirin and is non-ulcerogenic. Clopidogrel is free from most of the side effects of ticlopidine from which it was modified.

Surgical or procedural measures

Carotid artery stenosis

Internal carotid artery (ICA) stenosis (Figure 6.2) increases the risk of ISS via thromboembolic or haemodynamic mechanisms. The actual risk of stroke is increased by the following factors:

occurrence of symptoms (TIA or stroke), degree of stenosis, presence of ulceration, contralateral occlusion, inadequate collaterals, coexistence of other risk factors, and cerebral infarction on CT.

In asymptomatic patients, severe (70–99%) ICA stenosis carries a low risk of stroke (1.5–2% per year). Use of low-dose aspirin and modification of risk factors are recommended, since carotid endarterectomy can be complicated by stroke or death. In symptomatic cases (with TIA or ISS), severe ICA stenosis carries a high risk: for those with TIA, 12–13% rate of stroke in the first year and a cumulative rate of 30–35% in five years; for ISS, the respective risks are 5–9% and 25–45%. Carotid endarterectomy markedly reduces the risk of stroke to 1–3% per year, but should be carried out by experienced surgeons.

Percutaneous carotid angioplasty and stenting (Figure 6.2) is an alternative to carotid endarterectomy. Scenarios favouring angioplasty/stenting include anticipated high rate of peri-endarterectomy stroke or death, concomitant medical conditions, radiation-induced stenosis, and restenosis after endarterectomy.

Extracranial-to-intracranial (EC-IC) bypass

EC-IC bypass may restore blood flow to the cerebral hemisphere in patients with internal carotid artery occlusion or middle cerebral artery stenosis. However, the operation was shown to be ineffective in preventing stroke or death by the EC-IC Bypass Study.

7 Epilepsy

An epileptic seizure is a brief and usually unprovoked stereotyped disturbance of behaviour, emotion, motor function or sensation which on clinical evidence results from cortical neuronal discharge. Epilepsy, a disease rather than disorder, should only be diagnosed if one of the following conditions is met:

1. At least two unprovoked (or reflex) seizures occurring more than 24 hours apart
2. A single seizure with a high probability of further seizures, e.g., brain contusion, meningioma
3. Diagnosis of an epilepsy syndrome, e.g., juvenile myoclonic epilepsy

Under the new definition, epilepsy is considered 'resolved' for those who had an age-dependent epilepsy syndrome but are now past the applicable age or those who have remained seizure-free for the last 10 years and without use of AED for the last 5 years. Relapse is very rare after epilepsy has resolved.

Epidemiology and natural history

The prevalence of epilepsy is about 1 in 200–400. About 20–35% of cases are drug resistant. Recurrence occurs in about 60–80% of patients with a first idiopathic seizure and usually takes place within six months of the first attack.

Good prognostic factors include seizures precipitated by alcohol, drugs or metabolic disturbances, benign syndromes such as benign epilepsy with centrotemporal spikes and idiopathic generalized epilepsy. Poor prognostic factors include diffuse cerebral disorder (of which mental retardation is common), early onset seizures, recurrent seizures after onset of treatment, lesional epilepsies (e.g., hippocampal sclerosis, cortical dysplasia, and low-grade gliomas) and progressive neurological disorders (e.g., progressive myoclonic epilepsy and Lennox-Gastaut syndrome).

Standardized mortality rates are 2–3 times higher than those of the general population. The causes of death include accidents, status epilepticus, cerebrovascular disease, pneumonia, and suicide. Sudden deaths may be attributed to drowning, accidental asphyxia, neurogenic pulmonary oedema, and fatal cardiac arrhythmias. Sudden unexpected death in epilepsy (SUDEP) rarely occurs and its aetiology is unknown.

Aetiology

The age at onset usually provides some clues to the underlying cause (Table 7.1). In general, seizures are classified into reactive, idiopathic (primary), and symptomatic (secondary). Cryptogenic seizures are presumed to be symptomatic but the aetiology is unknown.

Table 7.1   Aetiology of seizures according to age at onset

Age (years)	Common causes
< 1	Hypoxia, hypoglycaemia, hypocalcaemia, kernicterus, birth trauma, intracranial haemorrhage, congenital anomalies
1–5	Intracranial infections, febrile seizures
5–20	Idiopathic epilepsy, head injury, cortical dysplasia, hippocampal sclerosis
20–60	Cerebral tumours, alcohol, drugs and toxins, CNS infections, AVM
> 60	CVD, neurodegenerative diseases, systemic illnesses, brain metastasis

Reactive seizures can be considered as a natural response of a relatively normal brain to insults such as alcohol withdrawal, head injury, and convulsing agents. Some normal subjects with a low seizure threshold may develop seizures with minor stress, such as sleep deprivation or emotional disturbance. AED prophylaxis is usually not required and the rational treatment is elimination of the precipitating factor(s).

The term 'idiopathic' implies the absence of structural brain lesions or neurological disorders. However, a genetic predisposition or occult biochemical defect is possible (e.g., chanelopathy). A positive family history is not uncommon and response to AED is generally satisfactory. Certain idiopathic epilepsies, both generalized and partial, are related to genetic defects. Examples are juvenile myoclonic epilepsy and autosomal dominant nocturnal frontal epilepsy syndrome. The age at onset is usually between 5 and 18 years. SCN1A mutations may give rise to a spectrum of genetic epilepsy ranging from generalized epilepsy with febrile seizure (GEFS) plus to Dravet syndrome (infantile myoclonic epilepsy).

Structural brain lesions and neurological dysfunction are frequently identified in symptomatic seizures, in which the risk of recurrence is high and the response to drug treatment less satisfactory.

Diagnosis of epilepsy

There are two levels of diagnosis: seizure type and underlying aetiology. Both have prognostic and therapeutic implications.

The patient's description of events and an eyewitness account are essential for diagnosis. Generalized seizures can be diagnosed with reasonable certainty in the presence of unconsciousness together with one or more of the following features: tonic-clonic convulsions, myoclonic jerks, tonic spasms, tongue biting, excess salivation, head turning, automatism, and a preceding aura. The aura is usually a psychic or somatic symptom such as fear, epigastric rising sensation, *déjà vu*, depersonalization or other forms of hallucinations. Post-ictal confusion or headache lasting for several hours is a useful pointer to epileptic seizures. The circumstances in which attacks occur, the preceding symptoms and precipitating factors are useful in differentiating seizures from non-epileptic conditions (Table 7.2).

The initial event also provides the best clue to the type of seizure and its origin. Typical auras are, strictly speaking, simple partial seizures and usually consistent for a given patient. Complex partial seizures (CPS) are characterized by a triad of aura, altered

Table 7.2 Differentiating features in epilepsy, syncope, and non-epileptic seizures

Clinical features	Syncope	Epilepsy	Psychogenic seizures
Onset	Gradual	Sudden	Variable, subtle
Associated symptoms	Giddiness, palpitations	Aura, prodrome	Inconsistent
Conscious level	Brief LOC (seconds)	LOC (minutes)	Prolonged LOC (hours)
Injury	Rare	Tongue biting	Rare
Complexion	Pale	Cyanosis	Usually no change
Convulsive jerk	Rare	Tonic or clonic	Asynchronous limb movements
Resist eye opening	Unusual	Unusual	Common
Incontinence	Rare	Common	Rare
Postictal confusion	Rare	Common	Often absent
Aggravating factors	Crowded places Unpleasant situations	Sleep deprivation Menstruation	Induced by suggestion or placebo injection
Ictal EEG	Diffuse slow waves	Epileptic discharges	Alpha rhythm with artefacts

LOC = loss of consciousness

consciousness and automatism. Ictal EEG recording shows that CPS arises not only from the temporal lobe, but also the frontal, parietal, and occipital lobe. Tracing partial seizures to the anatomical origin is essential in planning resective surgery. The differentiation between absence seizures and CPS is also important as their treatments are entirely different.

Differential diagnosis

1. Syncope
2. Hyperventilation syndrome
3. Transient ischaemic attack; transient global amnesia
4. Metabolic encephalopathy, e.g., hypoglycaemic attack, hepatic encephalopathy
5. Psychiatric conditions, e.g., panic attack, non-epileptic seizures
6. Movement disorders, e.g., paroxysmal choreoathetosis, hemifacial spasm, startle syndrome
7. Drop attacks without loss of consciousness
8. Sleep disorders, e.g., sleep walking, narcolepsy-cataplexy syndrome

Investigations

With the exception of hypoglycaemia, hypocalcaemia and hypomagnesemia, routine blood tests seldom provide clues to the aetiology. Leucocytosis and elevated CPK or prolactin may be evident after generalized tonic clonic seizures (GTCS). Neuroimaging may reveal a structural cerebral lesion amenable to surgery, e.g., glioma, meningioma or AVM. The chance of identifying a lesion is higher in partial seizures, in the presence of focal neurological signs and lateralized EEG abnormalities. In adult onset cases, MRI (or CT brain) should be routinely performed because of the increased likelihood of structural lesions. MRI is more sensitive in localizing lesions particularly for temporal lobe epilepsy. However, the lesion detected on neuroimaging may be coincidental and clinical correlation is essential.

EEG may provide evidence to support the diagnosis, aid classification, and suggest an aetiology, but its findings have to be interpreted in the clinical context. Inter-ictal EEG cannot confirm or exclude the diagnosis of epilepsy. About 10–15% of the population may have an 'abnormal' EEG which is of no diagnostic significance. More importantly, about 1% of the normal population have spikes and slow waves in the EEG. A single routine EEG is likely to show epileptiform activity in about 50% of patients with epilepsy. The chance of documenting an abnormal EEG is increased with repeated recording and sleep deprivation. Nevertheless, 15% of patients with epilepsy will not show epileptic features on inter-ictal EEG. The diagnostic yield can be enhanced with the use of prolonged video-EEG or ambulatory EEG recording. The former documented both ictal behaviour and EEG changes so that actual seizures can be recorded for semiology analysis, seizure classification and localization of epileptic focus. Two EEG records of epileptic discharges are shown in Figure 7.1 and Figure 7.2, which are of diagnostic and prognostic significance.

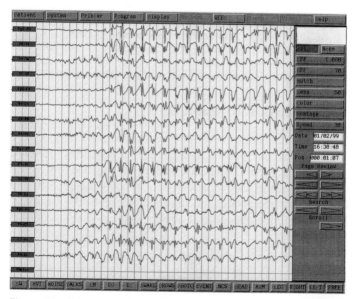

Figure 7.1 Scalp ictal EEG recording of absence seizures. The EEG demonstrates a short strip of normal recording followed by generalized high amplitude spike wave discharges at 3.5 Hz.

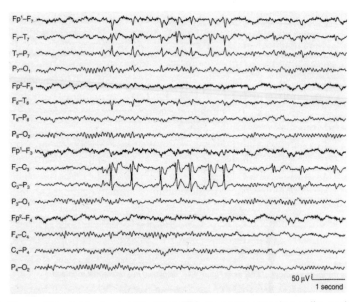

Figure 7.2   A bipolar longitudinal EEG montage showing spike and slow wave with phase reversal at C3 and T7. This is consistent with benign epilepsy with central temporal spikes (BECTS), a common partial epilepsy syndrome in children with good prognosis.

Classification of epilepsy

The current classification of epilepsy by ILAE takes into account not only seizure types but also the age at onset, EEG features, precipitating factors, anatomy, and aetiologic and prognostic factors. However, only about one-third of adult epilepsies fit into a 'diagnostic' category of epilepsy syndrome under this classification. A simplified and practical version of epilepsy classification is shown in Figure 7.3.

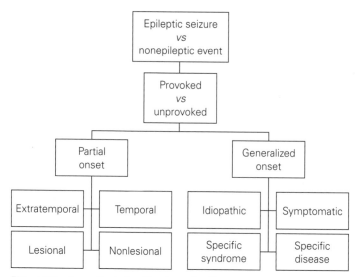

Figure 7.3   A practical classification of epilepsy.

Use of anti-epileptic drugs (AEDs)

Compliance with AEDs cannot be taken for granted. The side effects and the need to take long-term medication are deterrents. Careful explanation of the benefits and side effects of the AEDs would enhance patient's understanding and motivation. It is also helpful to let patients express their own views and feelings. Complete abolition of seizures with AED monotherapy can be achieved in 60% of patients and about 10% of patients respond to duo-therapy. Drug-resistant epilepsy occurs in about 20–30%. Treatment with three or more drugs is more likely to produce cognitive impairment and complicated drug interactions.

Starting AED treatment

The indications for commencing AED treatment are summarized in Table 7.3. The drug selected should be introduced slowly with a small starting dose, as too rapid an introduction may induce side effects resulting in non-compliance.

Table 7.3   Starting AED treatment

	Usual practice	Factors that may modify usual practice
Prospective risk of epilepsy	No treatment	Start AED for prophylaxis following head injury or surgery or in high risk conditions, e.g. AVM, brain tumour, SAH
Single seizure (clinically diagnosed)	No treatment	Progressive cerebral disorder Clearly epileptic EEG
Two or more seizures (clinically diagnosed)	Monotherapy	Withhold AED if: Seizures widely separated in time (> 1 year) Precipitating factors identified (e.g. alcohol, reflex stimuli, sleep deprivation) High probability of poor compliance (e.g. personality disorder)

Choice of AED

The choice of AED is based primarily on the seizure type (or epilepsy syndrome), patient characteristics and side effect profile of individual AEDs (Tables 7.4 and 7.5). First-line AEDs include carbamazepine, valproate, ethosuximide, and levetiracetam. Because of hirsuitism and gum hypertrophy, phenytoin is less often used than in the past, especially in women and children. Older AEDs including phenobarbitone, primidone and clonazepam should be avoided if possible in view of the sedative effect, and mild cognitive slowing on prolonged use.

Table 7.4 Choice of AED

Tonic-clonic or partial seizures	Simple absence seizure	Myoclonic seizures	Tonic, atonic, and atypical absence seizures	Lennox-Gastaute syndrome
Carbamazepine*	Valproate[+]	Valproate**	Valproate	Valproate
Oxcarbazepine	Ethosuximide[+]	Clonazepam	Carbamazepine	Clonazepam
Phenytoin*	Clonazepam	Clobazam	Phenytoin	Lamotrigine
Valproate[#]	Lamotrigine	Piracetam	Clonazepam	Vigabatrin
Lamotrigine		Levetiracetam	Phenobarbitone	Topiramate
Phenobarbitone			Clobazam	
Clobazam			Lamotrigine	
Primidone			Primidone	
Vigabatrin			Felbamate	
Gabapentin				
Topiramate				
Levetiracetam				
Pregabalin				

*   Drug of first choice for all tonic-clonic and partial seizures
[+]   Drug of first choice for simple absence seizures
[#]   Drug of first choice for primary generalized tonic-clonic seizures
**   Drug of first choice for myoclonic seizures

Table 7.5   Common adverse effects of AEDs

A. Standard AEDs	
• Carbamazepine	rash, hyponatraemia, drowsiness, drug interactions
• Valproate	weight gain, tremor, alopecia, teratogenicity
B. New AEDs	
• Oxcarbazepine	similar to carbamazepine but less enzyme induction
• Gabapentin	dizziness, somnolence
• Pregabalin	dizziness, ataxia, weight gain
• Lamotrigene	rash e.g., toxic epidermal necrolysis
• Levetiracetam	seizure exacerbation, dizziness
• Topiramate	paraesthesia, weight loss, cognitive slowing
• Vigabatrin	peripheral visual loss
• Lacosamide	dizziness, unsteadiness
• Perampanel	drowsiness, behavioural disturbance
C. Old AEDs	
• Phenytoin	rash, acne, facial coarsening, gum hypertrophy
• Phenobarbitone	sedation, cognitive slowing

AEDs marketed in or after the 1990s are known as new AEDs. They include gabapentin, oxcarbazepine, lamotrigene, vigabatrin, topiramate, levetiracetam, zonisamide, pregabalin, retigabine, lacosamide, and peranpanel. They have similar efficacy as standard AEDs but fewer side effects and drug interactions. They are often used as add-on treatment for drug-resistant epilepsy. They may also be used as monotherapy in selected patients, and are recommended if standard AEDs are contraindicated due to potential drug interaction (e.g., with oral contraceptives, anticoagulants) or unacceptable side effects.

Therapeutic drug monitoring (TDM)

The aim of AED therapy is control of seizures with minimal or no toxicity. Because efficacy and toxicity can often be assessed clinically with accuracy, and since these two parameters do not always have a consistent relationship with serum AED levels, routine monitoring of drug levels is not necessary for every patient.

It should also be emphasized that if a certain dose of an AED controls the epilepsy, a higher dose is not indicated even if the drug level is low.

The value of TDM lies in checking compliance, arriving at an individualized dose, keeping AED dose in step with body weight in growing children or during pregnancy, and avoiding drug intoxication. This is particularly so for phenytoin, the elimination of which follows saturation kinetics with a non-linear relationship between drug dose and plasma level. As the clearance of lamotrigine is greatly enhanced during the third trimester of pregnancy, TDM is useful in guiding the dosage and maintaining efficacy.

Side effects of AED

The most common CNS toxic effects of AEDs (except valproate and ethosuximide) are drowsiness and a cerebellar syndrome (slurred speech, nystagmus, limb and gait ataxia), but these can usually be avoided if there is no overdose or rapid dose escalation. Interaction with protein bound drugs (e.g., warfarin, oral contraceptives, other AEDs) usually occurs when a larger dose of AED is used. Such interaction should also be considered during AED withdrawal.

The side effects of AED may be more apparent or unacceptable in certain patient groups and such factors may influence the choice of AED.

1. Elderly: impaired drug clearance and increased susceptibility to side effects, e.g., hyponatraemia due to carbamazepine
2. Children: avoid phenobarbitone (behavioural disturbance) and phenyotin (cosmetic side effect and erratic absorption)
3. Reproductive women: avoid valproate (teratogenicity) and carbamazepine if oral contraceptives are required.
4. Professionals (cognitive slowing unacceptable): avoid phenobarbitone and topiramate.
5. Mental retardation: mood changes more common with topiramate; carbamazepine or valproate is preferred.
6. Uraemia: avoid gabapentin, which is mainly excreted by the kidney.

7. Active liver disease: avoid valproate (risk of hepatic encephalopathy).
8. HLA-B*1502 allele (present in 20% of Han Chinese) is associated with a dramatically increased risk of Stevens-Johnson syndrome. A positive test would suggest alternative AEDs other than carbamazepine

Stopping AED treatment

The risk of recurrence cannot be reliably determined. Hence, the medical and social implications (e.g., on driving and on employment) of recurrence should be weighed carefully against the side effects of long-term AED treatment (Table 7.6). In general, AED withdrawal is effected in 6 weeks to 3 months. Acute withdrawal is justified in case of severe complications, e.g., Stevens-Johnson syndrome; a benzodiazepine (e.g., clobazam) may be used as short-term cover to prevent withdrawal seizures.

Table 7.6   Stopping AED treatment

Absolute criteria	Factors in favour	Factors against
Two years free of seizures	Childhood epilepsy	Late onset epilepsy
Patient's informed consent	Primary generalized epilepsy except juvenile myoclonic epilepsy	Partial epilepsy except benign Rolandic epilepsy
	Idiopathic	Symptomatic
	Short duration of epilepsy	Long duration of epilepsy
	Normal EEG	Abnormal EEG
	Non-driver	Driver
	First remission	Previous relapse on withdrawal

Management of provoked seizures

Seizures may be provoked by metabolic disturbances, drug administration (e.g., imipenem), drug withdrawal (e.g., alcohol,

benzodiazepines), substance abuse, CNS infection (e.g., encephalitis), head injury, and stroke. Recurrence of such seizures can
be reduced by correction or withdrawal of the provoking factor.
Long-term AED therapy is usually not necessary. In severe head
injury and craniotomy, AED (e.g., IV valproate or levetiracetam)
may be used to prevent provoked seizures in the acute phase, but
prophylactic AED does not prevent subsequent development of
epilepsy.

General advice to patients with newly diagnosed epilepsy:
1. Avoid sleep deprivation.
2. Avoid prolonged television viewing or video games.
3. Avoid alcohol.
4. Avoid drugs which may lower seizure threshold, e.g., codeine,
   theophylline.
5. Dietary restriction is usually not necessary.
6. Alternative treatments, e.g., herbs, aromatherapy, and foot
   reflexology, may increase the risk of seizure.
7. Employ stress modification to restore psychological well-being.
8. Join epilepsy organizations for support.

Management of drug resistant epilepsy (DRE)

Modern treatment of epilepsy is effective for most patients,
as shown by the clinical course of 100 patients following treatment (Figure 7.4). Nevertheless, there is a significant proportion
of patients with DRE, which can be defined by failure to achieve
seizure remission for more than 12 months after adequate trials
of two appropriately selected AEDs (monotherapy or in combination). A full work-up or referral to epilepsy centres is often
required.
1. Look for precipitating factors of seizures, e.g., alcoholism, drug
   abuse, sleep deprivation, stress, and eliminate them if possible.
2. Check drug compliance and monitor AED levels.
3. Review the underlying cause. A progressive brain disorder
   (e.g., glioma) may have been overlooked.
4. Review the choice of AED in relation to the seizure type.

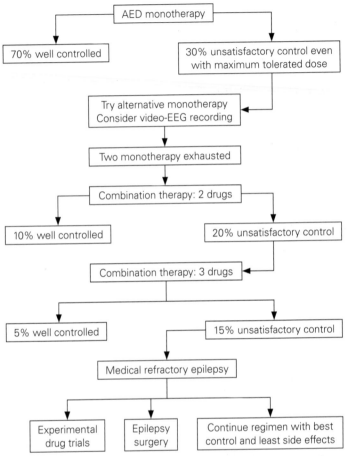

Figure 7.4 Expected outcome of AED treatment in 100 adult patients with epilepsy. Reproduced from 'Epilepsy: An Update on Diagnosis and Management', *Hong Kong Pract* 1996; 18(7): 322–330.

5. Consider the possibility of non-epileptic (psychogenic) seizures. Obtain a detailed account of attacks, explore the patient's psychological and social background, and refer to a psychiatrist if necessary. Non-epileptic seizures may coexist with genuine seizures in certain people with epilepsy.

6. If the patient cannot tolerate a first-line AED even at low dosages, replace the drug with another first-line AED. Otherwise, the dose should be increased slowly to the maximum tolerated amount. For AED substitution, the replacement should be added gradually before the ineffective one is slowly withdrawn.
7. Combination therapy can be initiated early for anticipated DRE.
8. Should a combination of two first-line agents prove unhelpful, the drug which appears to have greater efficacy and less side effects should be continued, while the other is replaced by a second-line AED.
9. Patients with true DRE should be referred for pre-surgical evaluation, trial of a new AED or other non-AED treatment.

Epilepsy surgery

Epilepsy surgery usually employs a resection or disconnection procedure aiming at eradication of seizures while sparing the functional cortex. Pre-surgical evaluation consists of a series of investigations to identify the epileptogenic zone and determine the adjacent cortical function. These tests include video-EEG recording ± invasive intracranial EEG, neuroimaging, WADA test to determine language lateralization and memory function of each temporal lobe, and cortical mapping. Proper selection of candidates is the key to success.

Lesional epilepsy constitutes the largest group of adult epilepsy for which surgery may offer a cure. Simple lesionectomy, if complete, can achieve a seizure remission rate comparable to formal epilepsy surgery. The underlying pathology and the completeness of lesion resection appear to be the two most important factors governing subsequent seizure remission.

Anterior temporal lobectomy is the standard surgical treatment for temporal lobe epilepsy, with a success rate of 70–80% worldwide. It often comprises excision of mesial temporal structures (including amygdala, hippocampal head and body, uncus, entorhinal region, the parahippocampal gyrus), and a variable portion of tip of temporal lobe. For extratemporal epilepsy, localization is much more difficult and often requires multimodal neuroimaging and intracranial EEG recording. Resection at eloquent region may not be possible because of unacceptable side effects, e.g., dysphasia and hemiplegia. Disconnection procedures (e.g., multiple subpial transection or corpus callosotomy) may be considered as palliative options.

Neurostimulation for DRE

Neurostimulation has expanded in scope substantially since 1997, starting with vagus nerve stimulation (VNS), followed by deep brain stimulation of the anterior thalamus, responsive neurostimulation and trigeminal nerve stimulation.

VNS is mainly indicated in DRE, which is not amenable to epilepsy surgery. Regular pulsed stimulation via the vagus nerve may desynchronize cerebral activity, enhance synthesis of inhibitory neurotransmitters, and hence reduce the risk of seizure. T-VNS involves transcutaneous stimulation of the auricular branch of the vagus nerve may turn out to be an equivalent non-invasive form of VNS.

The anterior nucleus of thalamus is a core component of the Papez circuit with close connection with the mesial temporal structures, and relay discharges for seizure spread. Inhibition of anterior thalamus via electrical stimulation may abort seizures in deep brain stimulation.

Women with epilepsy

Enzyme-inducing AEDs reduce the efficacy of oral contraceptives and high-dose oestrogen preparations may be necessary. Advice should be given on alternative means of contraception, and TDM may be necessary.

Since idiopathic generalized epilepsy may be familial, genetic counselling is required. If one parent has idiopathic epilepsy, the risk of epilepsy in the offspring is small; if both have epilepsy, the risk is increased (up to one in four).

Epilepsy should not preclude a woman from bearing and rearing children. If the patient fulfils the criteria for stopping AED, drug withdrawal may be offered before contemplating pregnancy. When treatment is necessary, monotherapy is preferred; polypharmacy carries a higher risk of congenital malformation. In most cases, the patient can be reassured of a satisfactory outcome.

All AEDs are weakly teratogenic and the overall frequency of congenital malformations is about 6% (3 times the background rate). However, stopping therapy and allowing seizures to recur in early pregnancy is harmful to both the mother and foetus. Carbamazepine has the least, if any, teratogenicity; reports of craniofacial defects, fingernail hypoplasia and developmental delay are largely anecdotal. Phenytoin may give rise to foetal-hydantoin syndrome. Valproate is known to produce neural tube defects and subsequent IQ decline at the age of 3, so switching to a safer AED appears justified for a planned pregnancy. If the patient is already pregnant, it is usually too late to switch AED because teratogenic effects occur in the first trimester. Folate supplement is recommended to all women with epilepsy during pregnancy. Teratogenicity data are limited for the new AEDs, and they should therefore be used with caution during pregnancy.

Since the metabolic elimination of most AEDs is increased during pregnancy, TDM may be necessary to assess the need for dosage increase e.g., lamotrigine. Accordingly, the dose should be decreased after delivery to avoid toxicity.

Most AEDs appear in the mother's milk during lactation, but not in quantities that affect the neonate. Mothers should be allowed to breast-feed if this is their wish. Neonatal sedation can result if the patient is receiving high doses of phenobarbitone or a ben-zodiazepine, in which case bottle feeding alternating with breast feeding should be tried.

Management of status epilepticus (SE)

SE is traditionally defined as seizures lasting more than 30 minutes, or several distinct episodes without restoration of consciousness. It is a neurological emergency which should be managed in the ICU. Most GTCS would terminate in 2–3 minutes and hence GTCS lasting longer than 5 minutes is likely to evolve into SE and hence deserves urgent treatment. Frequent seizures within a short period of time should also be regarded as SE and treated as such. Common causes of SE include abrupt withdrawal of AED in patients with known epilepsy, symptomatic epilepsy (e.g., CVD, brain tumours, anoxia and CNS infections), and metabolic disturbance (e.g., alcohol withdrawal, drug overdose, hepatic encephalopathy). SE can be classified according to seizure types (Table 7.7).

The mortality of SE was 50% prior to 1960 but has been reduced to 10% with modern ICU care. The outcome depends on the underlying aetiology and the time elapsed before initiation of treatment. Apart from permanent brain damage, possible complications following SE are listed in Table 7.8.

Table 7.7   Classification of status epilepticus

Generalized status	Partial epilepticus status	Non-epileptic status
Generalized tonic-clonic	Simple partial	Psychogenic
Generalized tonic	Complex partial	Decorticate posturing
Generalized clonic		Decerebrate rigidity
Generalized myoclonic		
Generalized absence		

Table 7.8   Systemic effects of status epilepticus

Cardiovascular	Hypotension, arrhythmia, sinus tachycardia
Respiratory	Apnoea, aspiration, pulmonary oedema
Renal	Rhabdomyolysis and renal failure
Metabolic	Acidosis, hyperkalaemia, hyponatraemia, hypoglycaemia
Autonomic	Hyperpyrexia, hyperhydrosis
Endocrine	Elevated prolactin, glucagon, growth hormone, adrenocorticotrophic hormone
Haematological	Leucocytosis, DIC
Skeletal	Orthopaedic injuries, fractures or dislocations

Initial management

1. Remove false teeth, establish a patent airway, and give oxygen by mask.
2. Assess the patient and place him/her in the left lateral position.
3. Give diazemuls or diazepam 10 mg IV bolus, followed by another 10 mg after 10 minutes if necessary.
4. Lorazepam 4 mg IV and midazolam IV/IM are alternatives to diazemuls/diazepam.
5. Check serum AED levels, glucose, electrolytes, alcohol, and toxicology.
6. Give 50 ml 50% glucose IV if haemoglucostix reveals low glucose.
7. Give thiamine 100 mg IV if alcoholism is suspected.
8. Give phenytoin 18 mg/kg IV (usually 1 g) at a rate of < 50 mg/ min.
9. To avoid possible cardiac side effects of phenytoin, IV valproate, IV levetiracetam, and IV lacosamide are useful alternatives.
10. In patients with known epilepsy, give the usual AEDs orally, via nasogastric tube or IV.
11. Do not leave the patient until seizures have stopped.
12. IV administration of diazepam may cause respiratory depression; therefore BP, ECG and oximeter monitoring during administration is desirable. Rectal diazepam 5–10 mg may be used as an alternative to IV route especially in children.
13. IV phenytoin is best given undiluted using syringe pump as it is highly alkaline and poorly soluble in dextrose solution; avoid extravasation which may produce thrombophlebitis.

Subsequent management

1. Transfer the patient to the ICU.
2. One of the following can be given:
    * Diazepam infusion at a rate of 5–10 mg/hr
    * Lorazepam (0.1 mg/kg) IV in 2–5 minutes

- Midazolam infusion (0.05–0.4 mg/kg/hr)
- Phenobarbitone (10 mg/kg) IV in 30 minutes; may be repeated after 12 hours
3. If seizures are not controlled within 2 hours, consult anaesthetist for general anaesthesia.
   - Thiopentone IV 5 mg/kg stat and maintained at 1–3 mg/kg/hr
   - Propofol IV 2 mg/kg stat and maintained at 0.2 mg/kg/min
   - Inhalational anaesthesia, isoflurane being the drug of choice
4. EEG monitoring is essential to determine whether there is ongoing seizure activity, especially in non-convulsive or subtle status epilepticus, and to monitor depth of anaesthesia.
5. Neuromuscular blockade alone does not prevent brain damage due to SE.
6. Maintenance AED therapy should be given, e.g., the dose of phenytoin is 5 mg/kg per day and that for phenobarbitone is 120–150 mg/day.
7. Ventilatory and cardiovascular support, adequate hydration, and treatment of infection are often necessary.
8. The cause of SE should be investigated and managed after the patient's condition is stabilized.

8 Movement Disorders

Movement disorders are neurological disorders which manifest as either excess movements (hyperkinesia, dyskinesia) or paucity of movements (bradykinesia, hypokinesia, akinesia). The different types of movement disorders include parkinsonism, tremor, chorea/choreoathetosis, tics, ballismus/hemiballismus, myoclonus, dystonia, and stiff-person syndrome.

The diagnosis is based primarily on the clinical picture since there is no diagnostic laboratory test in most cases. Video recording of the abnormal movements is helpful for difficult cases as this allows for post hoc analysis. Psychogenic movement disorder is not uncommon but should only be diagnosed after organic causes have been excluded.

Investigations should be directed by clues obtained from clinical examination. CT/MRI brain would be indicated if focal deficits are present. Serum copper and caeruloplasmin, urine copper and slit-lamp examination of the cornea should be considered in young patients with movement disorders. Other tests, including CBP, ESR, LFT, RFT, VDRL, heavy metal screening, genetic study, EEG, NCS, and EMG, are indicated in appropriate cases.

Parkinsonism

Clinical features

Parkinsonism is a clinical description of a movement disorder comprising rest tremor, rigidity, bradykinesia, and postural instability. Other clinical features include expressionless facies, loss of arm swing, dysarthria (typically monotonous speech), micrographia, dysphagia, drooling of saliva, constipation, autonomic dysfunction (including postural hypotension), conjunctivitis, vague aches, and pains.

Causes

- Idiopathic parkinsonism (Parkinson's disease) is the most common form.
- Secondary (symptomatic) parkinsonism
  - Postencephalitic, e.g., encephalitis lethargica, viral encephalitis
  - Drug-induced, e.g., neuroleptics, antihistamines, tetrabenazine
  - Toxic, e.g., manganese, carbon monoxide, 1-methyl-4-phenyl-1,2,3,6-tetrahydropyridine (MPTP), rotenone
  - Chronic head trauma, e.g., 'punch-drunk' syndrome
  - Neoplastic, e.g., parasagittal meningioma
- Parkinson-plus syndromes
  - Multisystem atrophy [MSA-pyramidal (MSA-P), MSA-cerebellar (MSA-C)])
  - Progressive supranuclear palsy (Steele-Richardson-Olzewski syndrome)
  - Corticobasal ganglionic degeneration (CBGD)
- Inherited neurodegenerative diseases
  - Wilson's disease
  - Neurodegeneration with brain iron accumulation (formerly known as Hallervorden-Spatz syndrome)
  - Familial olivopontocerebellar atrophy
- Pseudoparkinsonism
  - Cerebral arteriosclerotic disease
  - Normal pressure hydrocephalus

Differential diagnosis

As diagnosis of various forms of parkinsonism is made clinically, it can be difficult to differentiate other forms of parkinsonism from idiopathic parkinsonism. Even using strict diagnostic criteria, about 20% of patients with clinically definite Parkinson's disease may eventually be found to have other forms of parkinsonism.

The clinical features which are not typical of idiopathic parkinsonism include:

- Sudden onset of disease
- History of repeated strokes, with stepwise deterioration
- Frequent falls early in the disease
- Early dementia
- Early incontinence of faeces or urine
- No tremor in the presence of significant slowness of movement
- Gaze palsy
- Axial rigidity > limb rigidity
- Presence of pyramidal or cerebellar signs
- Poor response of symptoms to levodopa

Tremor

Tremor is the most common form of movement disorders (Table 8.1), and is characterized by rhythmical involuntary oscillatory movements which may affect the head, neck, voice, and limbs.

Diagnosis

A detailed history including the mode of onset, past health, drug and family history is important. Examine for other neurological features including focal deficits, cerebellar and extrapyramidal signs.

Treatment

Treat or remove any underlying cause. In physiological and essential tremor, propranolol, primidone, and benzodiazepines (e.g., clonazepam) can provide symptomatic relief. Cerebellar and rubral tremor do not respond well to drug treatment. Treatment of dystonic tremor and rest tremor are discussed in the sections on Dystonia and Parkinson's disease respectively.

Chorea/choreoathetosis

Chorea is characterized by sudden, unpredictable, involuntary, quasi-purposeful jerks. It is aggravated by voluntary movement, stress and anxiety, and disappears during sleep. It can be focal, lateralized or generalized.

Table 8.1   Types of tremor

Type of tremor	Causes and comments
Physiological tremor	Exaggerated in anxiety, thyrotoxicosis, chronic alcoholism, tremogenic drugs, e.g., neuroleptics, β_2-adrenoceptor agonists, calcium channel blockers, amiodarone, cyclosporine
Essential tremor	Typically presents as a postural tremor
Metabolic (flap) tremor	Carbon dioxide retention, hepatic or renal failure, mercury poisoning
Rest tremor	Predominantly in idiopathic parkinsonism
Kinetic tremor (occurs with movement)	Cerebellar tremor is the most frequent form of kinetic tremor. It occurs during voluntary movement and is characterized by jerky movements of the limb as it approaches the target (i.e., with intention)
	Task-specific tremor is most commonly encountered during handwriting. It may overlap with essential tremor.
Rubral or midbrain tremor	Low frequency tremor (3–5 Hz)
	Violent tremor due to lesions of red nucleus or its connections. It is a combination of postural and kinetic tremors. It occurs at rest, with posture and frequently exacerbated when approaching a target.
Dystonic tremor	Occurs in combination with dystonia
Psychogenic tremor	Variable frequency and amplitude, atypical pattern

Athetosis refers to slower, coarser, more writhing movements, especially affecting the distal parts of the limbs. Chorea frequently occurs together with athetosis (choreoathetosis).

Causes

- Drugs: neuroleptics, levodopa, dopamine agonists, antihistamines, amphetamines, digoxin, oral contraceptive pills
- Basal ganglia stroke
- Wilson's disease
- Sydenham's chorea
- Pregnancy (chorea gravidarum)
- Systemic illnesses: thyrotoxicosis, SLE, polycythaemia rubra vera, hypoparathyroidism, pseudohypoparathyroidism, neurosyphilis, kernicterus
- Huntington's disease
- Neuro-acanthocytosis
- Other neurodegenerative diseases (olivopontocerebellar atrophy, Pick's disease, neurodegeneration with brain iron accumulation, Creutzfeldt-Jakob disease)

Diagnosis

A detailed history including mode of onset, past health, drug history and family history is essential. A full neurological and cardiovascular examination together with slit-lamp examination of the cornea should be undertaken.

Treatment

Remove or treat any underlying cause. Tetrabenazine or clonazepam can be used for symptomatic control of chorea.

Ballismus/hemiballismus

Clinical features

The abnormal movements are similar to that of chorea but more severe in intensity. These consist of wild, flinging movements, usually involving the whole limb or one side of the body. In patients with vascular aetiology, they are usually sudden in onset and persist for a few weeks and then gradually subside.

Causes

As in chorea, ballismus can also be caused by a lesion in the contralateral subthalamic nucleus, e.g., stroke.

Treatment

Tetrabenazine is the drug of choice. Stereotactic thalamotomy may be carried out in unremitting cases.

Tics

Clinical features

Tics tend to be of childhood onset. They present as abrupt, jerky, and repetitive movements which involve discrete muscle groups. They can mimic normal coordinated movements, vary in intensity, lack rhythm (eye-blinks, head tossing, shoulder shrugs, facial grimaces), may be temporarily inhibited by will-power, and disappear during sleep. *Gilles de la Tourette's* syndrome occurs when tics are associated with vocalization including barks, grunts, and throat-clearing noises. Most cases resolve spontaneously after the age of 20 years.

Treatment

Response to drug therapy is in general unsatisfactory. Behavioural therapy is the mainstay of treatment. Reassurance to the family is essential.

Myoclonus

Clinical features

Myoclonus is characterized by brief, repetitive, sudden jerks involving a single muscle or muscle group(s). They appear like brief electric shocks which cannot be controlled by will-power. Myoclonus may persist during sleep, occur at rest, and be triggered by motor activity or other stimuli, e.g., touch, stretch.

Myoclonus is usually cortical (bilateral or generalized) in origin but can be non-cortical, e.g., in palatal myoclonus. Peripheral myoclonus is associated with spinal root, plexus or nerve lesions. Propriospinal myoclonus may be due to tumour, ischaemia or infection of the spinal cord.

Causes

- Exaggerated physiological myoclonus in startle syndromes, perinatal hypoxic encephalopathy, cocaine or amphetamine abuse
- Metabolic or toxic encephalopathies (due to cerebral anoxia, liver failure, renal failure, hyponatraemia, or hypoglycaemia)
- Progressive myoclonic epilepsy, mitochondrial encephalo-myopathy
- Neurodegenerative diseases, e.g., Creutzfeldt-Jakob disease, Alzheimer's disease, CBGD
- Metabolic storage diseases

Treatment

Treat the underlying cause if possible. Clonazepam, piracetam, and sodium valproate may provide symptomatic control.

Dystonia

It is a neurological syndrome dominated by involuntary muscle contractions which may be sustained, spasmodic or repetitive.

Classification

- Focal (a group of muscles), e.g., blepharospasm, oromandibular dystonia, cervical dystonia, writer's cramp, spasmodic dysphonia
- Segmental (contiguous group of muscles), e.g., craniobrachial dystonia, Meige syndrome
- Multi-focal (two or more non-contiguous groups of muscles)
- Generalized, e.g., idiopathic torsion dystonia

Clinical features

Contractions can affect any voluntary muscle. They are usually sustained such that affected body parts develop an abnormal posture. In the earlier stages, contractions tend to be worsened by voluntary action, fatigue, stress, and emotional states. However, they may be reduced with relaxation, hypnosis and 'sensory tricks' (frequently tactile and proprioceptive), and disappear during sleep. As dystonia progresses, it can occur at rest. Muscles involved tend to be hypertrophied. In later stages, fixed muscle contractures may develop. In primary dystonia, sensory, cerebellar or pyramidal deficits are usually absent, but voice tremor, or postural tremor of the limbs or head may be evident. Dystonia may progress to be more severe in the same body part or spread to other parts of the body. Patients who develop dystonia at a younger age tend to be more severely affected.

Mechanism

The pathophysiology of dystonia is unknown but may result from abnormal central motor processing of external sensory input.

Causes

- Idiopathic torsion dystonia. Hereditary forms begin in child-hood or early adolescence. They start in the lower limbs affecting the gait, spread rostrally and tend to become gener-alized. Inheritance may be autosomal dominant (AD), auto-somal recessive (AR) or X-linked. Sporadic forms are usually adult onset and symptoms are confined to upper limbs or axial structures.
- Secondary causes (especially in the presence of intellectual deterioration, pyramidal and extrapyramidal features, cerebel-lar ataxia, and sensory loss)
    - Parkinsonism
    - Cerebral palsy
    - Encephalitis
    - Drugs, e.g., neuroleptics, levodopa, metoclopramide, anti-histamines, methyldopa
    - Wilson's disease
    - Other neurodegenerative diseases, e.g., spinocerebellar ataxia, olivopontocerebellar atrophies, hereditary spastic paraplegia, neurodegeneration with brain iron accumulation, Huntington's disease
    - Metabolic storage diseases
    - Ataxia telangiectasia
- Pseudodystonia
    - Atlanto-axial subluxation
    - Stiff-person syndrome
    - Ligamentous/bony injury
    - Posterior fossa tumour
    - Psychogenic

Diagnosis

The diagnosis of dystonia depends on clinical examination. Video recording is helpful in documenting the dystonia and in monitor-ing progress.

Investigations are directed according to indications. In certain cases, additional investigations may include fresh blood smear for acanthocytes, lysosomal enzymes level in peripheral blood, arterial pH, serum lactate and pyruvate, urine collection for oligosaccharides, mucopolysaccharides, organic acids, and amino acids.

Treatment

- Specific therapy is aimed at treating specific causes, e.g., withdrawing the offending drug, commencing copper chelating therapy in Wilson's disease.
- Symptomatic treatment is aimed at maintaining function and reducing pain. It is not necessary to totally eliminate the dystonia. Most of the side effects of the drugs used in the treatment are dose-related.
  - Systemic pharmacotherapy: A small dose of levodopa should be tried initially in childhood-onset dystonia. In adult-onset cases, anticholinergic drugs and benzodiazepines (e.g., clonazepam) can be used.
  - Botulinum toxin is the therapy of choice in focal dystonias, and is also used in combination with systemic pharmacotherapy in segmental and generalized dystonia. Seven serotypes of toxin (A to G) are produced by *Clostridium botulinum*, but the most commonly used is Botulinum toxin-A. It is administered intramuscularly into affected muscles to relieve muscle spasms. It prevents the release of acetylcholine from the presynaptic nerve terminals at neuromuscular junctions and results in chemo-denervation of the muscle. Typically, its therapeutic effect starts in 24–72 hours and lasts 10–12 weeks. Botulinum toxin is generally safe but bruising, pain and stiffness can occur at the site of injection. Other side effects, e.g., muscle atrophy, weakness in injected muscles and in adjacent muscles, may occur. Dysphagia, ptosis, lower facial muscle weakness, and increased lacrimation may also develop depending on the site of injection. These side effects are reversible with reduced dosage or cessation of the drug.

SELECTED ENTITIES

Parkinson's disease (PD)

Its prevalence in the general population is about 3/1000. The elderly is mainly affected and onset before the age of 40 years is rare. The characteristic pathological changes are selective destruction of dopaminergic nigrostriatal neurons (resulting in cell loss and loss of neuromelanin) and Lewy bodies (eosinophilic intraneuronal inclusion bodies) within the neurons of the substantia nigra and locus coeruleus. Although families with parkinsonism are uncommon, mutated genes have been linked to these families.

The diagnosis is made by clinical examination. The features consist of rest tremor (4–6 Hz), cogwheel rigidity, bradykinesia and postural instability. These features tend to be more prominent on one side of the body especially in the early stages. Certain drugs (e.g., metoclopramide, antihistamines, phenothiazines) may aggravate the symptoms. It is important to exclude Wilson's disease in young patients and drug-induced parkinsonism. In patients with atypical features, MRI/CT brain should be considered.

Treatment

At present, there is no cure for this disease. The aim is to relieve parkinsonian symptoms with an individually tailored regime of medications so that the patient can maintain a normal lifestyle.

Drug therapy

Different categories of drugs are available.

Levodopa-based

Levodopa + carbidopa = Sinemet
Levodopa + benserazide = Madopar

Levodopa is the most efficacious drug available. It acts by replacing the reduced dopamine supply. It is decarboxylated to dopamine, which then acts on dopamine receptors in the corpus striatum. Dopa-decarboxylase inhibitors (carbidopa and benserazide) cannot pass the blood-brain-barrier and hence only prevent the peripheral decarboxylation of levodopa. This reduces excess dopamine formation outside the CNS (hence reducing peripheral side effects), and increases the bioavailability of levodopa to the brain.

Side effects: nausea, postural hypotension, confusion, agitation, and psychotic manifestations (e.g., delusions and hallucinations) are dose-related. At a later stage, motor fluctuations (e.g., 'wearing-off', 'on-off' phenomena, freezing), dyskinesias (peak-dose, biphasic), and akathisia occur in most patients.

Motor fluctuations typically progress from the early 'wearing-off' phenomenon (occasionally as early morning akinesia), 'end-of-dose' deterioration, predictable 'off' periods, unpredictable 'off' periods, and eventually to unpredictable 'on-off' phenomenon in the advanced stage. Short-lived freezing episodes lasting seconds or minutes occur in the later stages of the disease.

Levodopa-induced dyskinesias usually comprise a mixture of chorea (sometimes ballismus) and dystonia. 'Peak-dose' dyskinesia (the most common type) initially responds to dose reduction. Later, dyskinesias occur at the 'on-off' interface and eventually the relationship of dyskinesias to the timing of levodopa dose becomes unclear and unpredictable. Akathisia bears no relationship to levodopa dosage and can occur in the 'on' or 'off' stage.

Measures to control motor fluctuations and dyskinesias include:
- Document motor fluctuations and dyskinesias on a chart.
- Low-protein diet (of limited effect)
- Tailoring of levodopa dosage to patient's activities
- Levodopa dose-fractionation
- Intraduodenal infusion of levodopa
- Addition of dopamine agonists (including apomorphine to control 'off' periods)

Dystonia can be eased with anticholinergic drugs or clonazepam.

Dopamine agonists

Examples include pramipexole, ropinirole, apomorphine, and rotigotine (administered via skin patch). They act directly on striatal dopamine receptors. Although less efficacious than levodopa, they are useful on their own at early stages of the disease especially for younger-onset patients. They are also used in combination with levodopa at later stages.

Side effects: nausea, vomiting, postural hypotension, headache, confusion, agitation, depression, hallucinations, and increase in dyskinesias

Monoamine oxidase-B inhibitors

Examples include selegiline (L-deprenyl) and rasagiline. They act by reducing dopamine oxidation and hence prolonging synaptic action of dopamine. It may be used as an adjunct to levodopa therapy, especially in younger-onset patients.

Side effects: insomnia, skin rash

Anticholinergic drugs

Examples are orphenidrine, benzhexol, and benztropine. They block muscarinic cholinergic fibres in the striatum. They are used in younger-onset patients especially those with prominent dystonia and tremor, or as an adjunct to levodopa.

Side effects: dry mouth, blurred vision, urinary retention, confusion, memory loss, and psychosis.

Amantadine

The exact mechanism of action is unclear but one of its anti-parkinsonian effects relies on N-methyl-D-aspartic acid (NMDA) receptor blockade.

Side effects: livedo reticularis, ankle oedema, poor concentration, dizziness, agitation

Catechol-O-methyltransferase (COMT) inhibitor-Entacapone

It is ineffective on its own and has to be prescribed with levodopa and dopa-decarboxylase inhibitor. It acts by reducing the methylation of dopamine (prolonging the synaptic action of dopamine) and levodopa (reducing the formation of plasma 3-O-methyldopa). High plasma 3-O-methyldopa (major metabolite of levodopa) concentration is associated with reduced efficacy of levodopa and levodopa-induced dyskinesias.

Side effects: dyskinesia, urine discolouration, diarrhoea

Physiotherapy and occupational therapy

Physical exercise to maintain body musculature and mobility should be encouraged. Specific measures, e.g., walking aids, use of chairs with straight back and arm rests, can help patients cope with daily life.

Surgical procedures

Drug therapy is symptomatic and is for life. Levodopa replacement is associated with reduced efficacy and motor fluctuations after 5–10 years of treatment.

Neurosurgery is beneficial in selected cases of Parkinson's disease. Surgical interventions include thalamotomy, pallidotomy, and chronic deep brain stimulation of globus pallidus or subthalamic nuclei. Thalamotomy is mainly used for control of medically intractable tremor. Pallidotomy may be used for control of levodopa-induced dyskinesias, rigidity, bradykinesia, and tremor. Chronic deep brain stimulation produces the same effects as permanent lesioning, but its effects disappear when stimulation ceases. Bilateral stimulation of the subthalamic nuclei appears to produce the best results.

Non-motor features

PD does not only manifest in motor disabilities, but also in non-motor features (Table 8.2). Motor disability is predominantly due to degeneration of dopaminergic nigrostriatal neurones. However, the neurodegenerative changes in PD is much more widespread involving non-dopaminergic neurones in cholinergic, noradrenergic, serotonergic, and GABAnergic pathways. Some non-motor features such as hyposmia, constipation, rapid eye movement sleep behaviour disorder, and depression may manifest even before the onset of motor features. Non-motor features can cause significant morbidity in PD, and are major determinants in its outcome. PD-dementia and PD-psychosis in advanced stages of the disease are common determinants for long-term nursing home care.

Table 8.2   Non-motor features

Neuropsychiatric disorders
Depression, apathy
Anxiety
PD-dementia
PD-psychosis

Autonomic dysfunction
Postural hypotension
Increased sweating
Urinary dysfunction
Sexual dysfunction
Constipation
Delayed gastric emptying, nausea

Sleep disorders
REM sleep behaviour disorder
Insomnia, fragmented sleep
Excessive daytime somnolence

Others
Hyposmia
Fatigue

PD-dementia develops in 10–15% of patients, especially in older-onset patients. It is worsened by anticholinergic therapy. Acetycholinesterase inhibitors (e.g., rivastigmine, donepezil) are used to reduce cognitive impairment.

Depression occurs in over 50% of patients. It is associated with serotonergic deficiency, which may not be relieved by levodopa or dopamine agonists. Antidepressants including selective serotonin reuptake inhibitors (e.g., citalopram, fluoxetine) are helpful.

PD-psychosis is relatively common in late stages of the disease. It can start as frightening nightmares, vivid dreams or illusions, and may progress to overt mania, hallucinations (usually visual) or delusions. It is often worsened by anticholinergics or dopamine agonists. Some atypical antipsychotics (e.g., quetiapine) are effective in ameliorating such features and do not usually aggravate the parkinsonian symptoms.

Anxiety is a common problem but is often left untreated. Benzodiazepines (e.g., diazepam, clonazepam) may be helpful.

Postural hypotension, if severe, gives rise to dizziness and falls. As levodopa or dopamine agonists may worsen this problem, the dosage may be reduced. Other measures include sleeping in a head-up tilt position, increasing salt intake, and small doses of fludrocortisone (in severe cases).

Constipation is common but often left untreated. Contributory factors include delayed bowel transit time inherent in Parkinson's disease, lack of exercise, and lack of fluid and fibre intake. A combination of a high-fibre diet, bulk-forming laxatives (e.g., metamucil), osmotic laxatives (e.g., lactulose), increased fluid intake and exercise are helpful. Bowel opening may be easier during an 'on period'. Short courses of stimulant laxatives (e.g., senokot, bisacodyl) may be required in more severe cases.

Increased sweating may result in seborrheic dermatitis over the scalp, face and trunk. This problem may respond to levodopa. Ichthammol lotions and shampoos containing selenium sulphide or zinc pyrithione may be helpful.

Parkinson-plus syndromes

Multisystem atrophy (MSA)

This group of disorders include MSA-pyramidal (MSA-P) and MSA-cerebellar (MSA-C), which account for up to 10% of parkinsonian patients. The pathology is characterized by widespread oligodendroglial tangle-like inclusions in the white matter, associated with degeneration within the subcortical nuclei especially in the substantia nigra and the striatum.

In addition to extrapyramidal features, other clinical features are present. These include pyramidal (MSA-P) and cerebellar (MSA-C) features, autonomic and urinary dysfunction. The age of onset is usually in the early 50s. An onset age of less than 30 years, a family history of the disorder or overt dementia are unusual in MSA.

Some patients with MSA may experience brief improvement following levodopa treatment. Fludrocortisone may be useful in patients with significant postural hypotension.

Progressive supranuclear palsy (Steele-Richardson-Olzewski syndrome)

It typically presents as parkinsonism with early loss of postural reflexes resulting in frequent falls. Supranuclear gaze palsy (primarily downwards) is characteristic, but oculocephalic responses are normal. Axial rigidity may predominate over limb rigidity. Dysarthria and dysphagia present early. Cognitive abnormalities particularly affect frontal lobe functions, e.g., personality change, progressive memory impairment, and uncontrolled emotional expression.

Response to levodopa is poor and the disease is progressive. Tricyclic antidepressants may be given for depression. Death often occurs within 6 years of onset, usually from pneumonia.

Corticobasal ganglionic degeneration (CBGD)

This disorder combines parkinsonian features with cortical dysfunction. The parkinsonian features which consist of postural tremor and instability, akinesia, limb rigidity, and dystonia are typically asymmetrical. Cortical signs associated with asymmetrical frontoparietal cortical atrophy include frontal release signs, apraxia, cortical sensory loss, and 'alien hand' syndrome. Other features include myoclonus, ocular gaze palsy, athetosis, dysphagia, dysarthria, and dementia.

Treatment is supportive. Clonazepam may be useful for myoclonus. Response to levodopa is poor. Death usually occurs from aspiration pneumonia.

Drug-induced movement disorders

Drugs can cause a variety of movement disorders. The most common offending drugs are neuroleptics, antihistamines and metoclopramide. Pre-existing CNS conditions, e.g., parkinsonism and previous Sydenham's chorea are significant predisposing factors.

Akathisia

Akathisia is a subjective desire to move, resulting in restlessness and inability to stand or sit still. It may be associated with dysphoric burning sensation. There are numerous abnormal stereotypic motor behaviours, e.g., criss-crossing of legs, wringing of hands, and rocking motion of the trunk. It is usually associated with exposure to more potent neuroleptics. It may occur within hours of first exposure and is believed to be due to blockade of mesocortical dopamine receptors.

Treatment

Anticholinergics, benzodiazepines, propranolol

Acute dystonic reactions

Acute dystonia including oculogyric crisis may develop within 48 hours of exposure to dopamine receptor blocker (e.g., haloperidol, metoclopramide). It tends to affect children and younger males.

Treatment

Anticholinergics (e.g., benztropine) and diphenhydramine are effective in relieving the symptoms.

Drug-induced parkinsonism

These individuals may have a predisposition to parkinsonism which might not have manifested at the time of exposure to the causative drug.

Treatment

Withdraw offending drugs. Levodopa or anticholinergic therapy may be used if parkinsonism persists despite withdrawal of the offending agent. If continuing neuroleptic therapy is required, an atypical neuroleptic (e.g., quetiapine) may be used.

Tardive dyskinesia

It is the most common movement disorder associated with long-term exposure to neuroleptics. It is believed to be due to striatal dopamine receptor supersensitivity. Tardive dyskinesia tends to occur in the elderly, females, and patients with affective disorders.

Clinical features

Movements are rhythmic and stereotyped. The most common manifestation is bucco-lingual-masticatory dyskinesia (complex chewing and tongue popping movements which can be rapid). It may also affect the extremities ('piano-playing' fingers) and trunk (body rocking). Parkinsonism may develop concomitantly. The disorder may be permanent. Paradoxically it may be worsened by withdrawal and suppressed by increased dosage of the offending drug. Once established, the natural history is variable. It usually attains its maximum severity rapidly before stabilizing.

Treatment and prognosis

Treatment is difficult. The offending drug can be withdrawn gradually. An atypical neuroleptic (e.g., quetiapine) may be used as a substitute. Tetrabenazine may offer symptomatic relief. Up to half of the patients may be in remission from tardive dyskinesia after prolonged withdrawal of the offending drug.

Neuroleptic malignant syndrome (see Chapter 16)

Essential tremor

It is the most common tremor for which people seek medical attention and can occasionally be confused with tremor of PD. It is typically an AD disorder but debate still exists as to whether it is a specific disease entity, symptom or syndrome.

Clinical features

The frequency of tremor usually ranges from 6–9 Hz. Typically, it presents as a postural tremor which becomes more pronounced during action or sustained postures. It usually affects the hands, head (titubation) or voice. The tremor can be disabling but may improve with alcohol consumption.

Treatment

Propranolol is indicated in symptomatic patients, and primidone and benzodiazepines are alternatives. In medically intractable cases, bilateral chronic deep brain stimulation of the ventral intermedius nucleus of the thalamus has been shown to be helpful.

Hemifacial spasm

Hemifacial spasm is characterized by involuntary twitching or spasms that contort the muscles innervated by the facial nerve on one side of the face. The chronic paroxysmal contractions have variable intensity, rhythm, and distribution. The spasms almost always start in adulthood and can be disabling. They may be precipitated by active movement of the facial muscles and fatigue, and may persist during sleep. It is idiopathic in most cases, but in a small percentage of patients, it may be associated with neurovascular contact of the facial nerve with blood vessels adjacent to the brainstem (shown on MRI). EMG shows that these spasms are due to high frequency discharges from motor units of the facial nerve.

Treatment

Injection of botulinum toxin into affected muscles is safe and efficacious. The response begins within a week and lasts for several months. Repeated injections are usually required for symptomatic control. Microvascular decompression of the affected facial nerve may be helpful, but this can be associated with greater risks including deafness postoperatively.

Wilson's disease

It is an AR multisystem disorder due to impaired incorporation of copper into caeruloplasmin and impaired biliary copper excretion, leading to deposition of copper in the brain (especially basal ganglia), liver, renal tubules, and cornea. It is associated with mutations in ATP7B, a copper-transporting ATPase.

Clinical features

Extrapyramidal features such as progressive dystonia, rigidity, bradykinesia, dysarthria, and tremor are common presenting features. In children, hepatic dysfunction (acute hepatitis and cirrhosis) tends to be prominent. Other features include acute haemolytic anaemia, biliary colic, arthritis, and seizures.

Diagnosis

It is suspected in the presence of progressive extrapyramidal signs (especially in young persons) and Kayser-Fleischer (KF) rings. Laboratory results including abnormal serum liver biochemistry, low serum copper and caeruloplasmin, and high 24-hour urinary copper excretion are confirmatory. In some cases, a liver biopsy is required for diagnosis.

Treatment

Treatment in the early symptomatic stage or in the asymptomatic phase of the disease provides the best outcome. There may be an initial deterioration of symptoms when treatment commences.

- D-penicillamine is used to remove excess copper. Pyridoxine supplement is also given because of the anti-pyridoxine effect of penicillamine. Triethylene tetramine dihydrochloride (trientine) can be used if D-penicillamine is not tolerated or causes unacceptable side effects.
- Low copper diet and zinc sulphate are used to prevent copper reaccumulation in the maintenance phase of treatment or in pre-symptomatic individuals.
- Liver transplantation is reserved for young patients with severe hepatic damage. Reversal of neurological impairment is possible.
- Treatment is monitored by clinical status, 24-hour urinary copper excretion, serum caeruloplasmin, serum liver biochemistry and slit-lamp examination.

Screening of family members

Screening of patient's first-degree relatives is mandatory. This process should include a detailed history and examination, slit-lamp examination of the eyes, serum liver biochemistry, caeruloplasmin level, and 24-hour urinary copper level. Affected relatives who are asymptomatic should undergo treatment as for affected individuals.

Huntington's disease

Huntington's disease is an AD disorder with the mean age at onset being 40 years old. The abnormal gene (Huntingtin, formerly known as IT15) has an expanded segment of CAG trinucleotide repeats that is unstable when transmitted to the next generation, changing in length during gamete formation. The pathology is characterized by atrophy of caudate and putamen with loss of medium spiny neurones.

Clinical features

The phenotype and age at onset can vary widely even within a given family. Juvenile-onset disease is the most disabling and is usually inherited from the father. Chorea is increased with stress and walking, and disappears during sleep. Psychiatric manifestations, e.g., chronic atypical depressive state, psychosis, disordered emotional states, are common. Cognitive abnormalities are frequently evident at the onset of chorea, e.g., deficits in planning, execution of complex tasks, attention and concentration. Dementia develops at a later stage. Other manifestations include dysarthria, dysphagia, and apraxia.

The disorder is progressive and is usually fatal within 10–15 years.

Diagnosis

The diagnostic features are the presence of chorea, cognitive deficits and family history. Identification of the mutant gene is confirmatory.

Treatment and prognosis

There is no effective treatment. Multidisciplinary care (e.g., psychological counselling, community care) is beneficial. Clonazepam or tetrabenazine may provide symptomatic control of chorea. Antidepressants, benzodiazepines, and phenothiazines are used to control depression, anxiety, and psychosis respectively. Relatives of affected patients require counselling, particularly if they wish to undergo the genetic test for the mutant gene.

9 Demyelinating Diseases of the Central Nervous System

Demyelinating diseases of the central nervous system (CNS) include multiple sclerosis (MS), acute disseminated encephalomyelitis (ADEM), neuromyelitis optica spectrum disorders (NMOSD), transverse myelitis, and central pontine myelinolysis. The bulk of damage lies in the white matter but grey matter may also be affected. The site, extent, and severity of demyelination, axonal injury, and grey matter involvement vary. The aetiology is heterogeneous.

SELECTED ENTITIES

Multiple sclerosis

MS is a disease of unknown aetiology primarily affecting the CNS. The lesions appear at different times and are disseminated in the spinal cord, optic nerve, brainstem, cerebellum and cerebrum. It is common in Caucasians but much less so in Orientals. There is a female preponderance (females to males = 3 to 1). Familial occurrence is rare in Orientals but not uncommon in Caucasians.

Clinical features

The first symptoms of MS usually occur between 15 and 55 years of age, and the average age of onset is 30 years. Accumulation of residual deficits from repeated episodes of demyelination and axonal injury eventually leads to significant loss of functional capacity. Typically in an unselected cohort, about 50% of patients have mild disability, 25% have moderate disability, and 25% have severe disability. Kurtzke Expanded Disability Status

Scale (EDSS) (Table 9.1) is commonly used to assess functional status. Recent studies have shown that subclinical attacks (with lesions detected on MRI) are much more common than clinical attacks. This observation is consistent with a chronic inflammatory process. MS can be classified into four clinical forms:

- Relapsing and remitting MS (RRMS)
  - most common form (85–90% of patients)
  - recovering clinically from individual attacks of demyelination
  - new clinical relapses unpredictable
- Secondary progressive MS (SPMS)
  - second most common form
  - in around 50% of the RRMS patients after about 15 years
  - variable progressive course without relapses and remissions
- Primary progressive MS (PPMS)
  - in about 10–15% of patients
  - variable progressive course from the beginning
- Progressive relapsing MS (PRMS)
  - in about 5% of patients
  - relapses superimposing on a progressive course

Table 9.1   Expanded Disability Status Scale (EDSS)

Disability in eight functional systems (FS)	Step
Normal neurological examination	0.0
No disability, minimal signs in one FS	1.0
No disability, minimal signs in more than one FS	1.5
Minimal disability in one FS	2.0
Mild disability in one FS or minimal disability in two FS	2.5
Fully ambulatory but with moderate disability in one FS or mild disability in three or four FS	3.0
Fully ambulatory but with moderate disability in one FS and more than minimal disability in several others	3.5
Fully ambulatory without aid, self-sufficient, up and about 12 hours a day despite relatively severe disability; able to walk without aid or rest some 500 metres	4.0
Fully ambulatory without aid, up and about much of the day, able to work a full day despite relatively severe disability; some limitation of full activity or requiring minimal assistance; able to walk without aid or rest some 300 metres	4.5

Table 9.1   (continued)

Disability in eight functional systems (FS)	Step
Ambulatory without aid or rest for 200 metres; disability severe enough to impair full daily activities	5.0
Ambulatory without aid or rest for 100 metres; disability severe enough to preclude full daily activities	5.5
Intermittent or unilateral constant assistance (cane, crutch, brace) required to walk 100 metres with or without rest	6.0
Constant bilateral assistance (canes, crutches, braces) required to walk 20 metres without rest	6.5
Unable to walk beyond 5 metres even with aid, essentially restricted to wheelchair; wheels self in standard wheelchair and transfers alone; up and about in wheelchair 12 hours a day	7.0
Unable to take more than a few steps; restricted to wheelchair; may need aid in transfer; wheels self but cannot carry on in standard wheelchair a full day; may require motorized wheelchair	7.5
Essentially restricted to bed or chair but out of bed much of the day; retains many self-care functions; has effective use of arms	8.0
Essentially restricted to bed much of the day; retains some self-care functions; has some effective use of arms	8.5
Confined to bed; can communicate and eat	9.0
Totally helpless and bed-bound; unable to communicate and eat	9.5
Death due to MS	10.0

Common presenting symptoms include visual loss, sensory, motor and/or cerebellar disturbances in the limbs. The distinctive features of MS include:
- Bilateral internuclear ophthalmoplegia
- Lhermitte's phenomenon (neck flexion giving rise to an electric shock sensation down the body)
- Sensitivity to heat (Uhthoff's phenomenon) with sensory, motor, or visual disturbance
- Unilateral optic neuritis

In addition, the common features are:

- Fatigue
- Nystagmus
- Trigeminal neuralgia
- Facial myokymia
- Brown-Séquard syndrome
- Transverse myelitis (short, partial)
- Hemiparesis, limb spasms
- Cerebellar ataxia
- Detrusor sphincter dyssynergia
- Sexual dysfunction
- Cognitive impairment

Diagnosis

Traditional diagnostic criteria of MS require at least two clinical relapses referable to separate CNS sites. When clinical evidence is insufficient to establish the diagnosis, radiological and laboratory findings are considered. MRI is the most sensitive tool in demonstrating lesions disseminated in space and in time (Figure 9.1a). MS lesions typically involve the periventricular white matter, corpus callosum, brainstem, and juxtacortical regions. One or more lesions in at least two of the four regions (e.g., periventricular, juxtacortical, infratentorial, spinal cord) are indicative of dissemination in space. As a result of breakdown of the blood-brain-barrier, acute lesions enhance with gadolinium (a paramagnetic contrast agent) on MRI. The presence of both acute enhancing lesions and old non-enhancing lesions is suggestive of dissemination of lesions in time. Since other disorders can cause lesions on MRI which meet the diagnostic criteria for MS, careful exclusion of such disorders is essential.

Positive CSF oligoclonal bands (OCB) or markedly prolonged VEP would also support the diagnosis of MS.

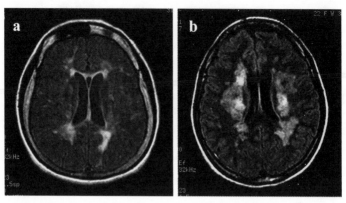

Figure 9.1 Fluid-attenuated inversion recovery (FLAIR) MRI brain images showing (a) multiple subcortical and periventricular hyperintense lesions in the white matter with involvement of the corpus callosum in MS, and (b) multiple patchy asymmetric subcortical hyperintense lesions of in the white matter of ADEM.

Variants of MS

- Balo's concentric sclerosis
- Marburg's variant
- Schilder's disease (myelinoclastic diffuse sclerosis)

Differential diagnosis

- Other demyelinating disorders, e.g., NMOSD, ADEM, transverse myelitis, central pontine myelinolysis
- Collagen vascular diseases, e.g., SLE, Sjögren's syndrome, PAN
- Primary CNS vasculitis
- Infections, e.g., neurosyphilis, HIV-1, Lyme disease, HTLV-1, PML
- Granulomatous diseases, e.g., sarcoidosis
- Vitamin B_{12} deficiency
- Genetic disorders, e.g., adult metachromatic leukodystrophy
- Endocrine disturbance, e.g., thyroid and adrenal disease
- Paraneoplastic encephalomyelitis

Treatment of acute attacks

Corticosteroid therapy is effective in reducing the duration and severity of acute exacerbations but has no significant effect on the functional outcome. Corticosteroids may alter the clinical course of optic neuritis and reduce disability in SPMS. Beneficial effects may include decreased blood-brain-barrier permeability, blockage of release of tumour necrosis factor, reduced activation of macrophages and lymphocytes, and decreased intrathecal production of immunoglobulins. Symptoms of progressive motor weakness, gait ataxia, limb ataxia, ophthalmoparesis, and vertigo are generally responsive to corticosteroids, whereas sensory symptoms are refractory. High dose (pulse) IV methylprednisolone followed by a tapering course of oral prednisolone is effective. Acute relapse without significant neurological recovery after pulse methylprednisolone may improve with plasmapheresis (7 exchanges in 2 weeks). Intensive physiotherapy is useful and may augment neurological recovery.

Prophylactic treatment with disease modifying therapy (immunomodulatory or immunosuppressive medications)

First line DMT

- Interferon beta
  - available as Interferon beta-1b (Betaferon) and Interferon beta-1a (Rebif and Avonex)
  - reduces the relapse rate and decreases new MRI lesions by inhibition of the effects of interferon gamma and monocytes, and down-regulation of T-cell functions
  - slows down long-term progression of physical disability and brain atrophy in RRMS and is also useful in SPMS
  - side effects include injection site reactions, flu-like illness, fever, myalgia, and systemic reactions (flushing, chest pain, palpitation, anxiety, dyspnoea)

- Glatiramer acetate (copolymer-1)
  - synthetic random copolymer of amino acids constituting myelin basic protein
  - suppresses experimental allergic encephalomyelitis (an animal model of MS)
- Teriflunomide (oral)
  - active metabolite of leflunomide, inhibitor of dihydroorotate dehydrogenase (a key mitochondrial enzyme for de-novo pyrimidine synthesis required by rapidly dividing B and T cells)
  - reduces relapse rate and slow disability progression
  - teratogenic
- Dimethyl fumarate (oral)
  - uncertain mechanisms, possesses anti-inflammatory and anti-oxidant properties mediated through activation of the nuclear factor (erythroid-derived 2)-like 2 (Nrf2) transcriptional pathway
  - reduces relapse rate, MRI disease activity and disability progression in RRMS
  - flushing and gastrointestinal symptoms are common side effects. Severe lymphopenia and PML may rarely occur.

Second line DMT

- Fingolimod (oral)
  - a sphingosine-1-phosphate (S1P) analogue which modulates S1P receptor and inhibits egress of lymphocytes from lymph nodes
  - reduces relapse rate and MRI disease activity, and slows down disability progression
  - adverse effects include first-dose bradycardia and heart-block, severe lymphopenia, VZV infection, and maculopathy.
  - needs immunization with VZV vaccine if seronegative for VZV IgG before initiation
  - teratogenic, strict contraception needed during therapy

- Natalizumab (monthly IV infusion)
  - monoclonal antibody against α4-integrin, prevents lymphocytes migration from peripheral blood into CNS
  - reduces relapse rate and MRI disease activity, and decreases risk of sustained disability progression
  - PML, an opportunistic infection of oligodendrocytes by JC virus, is the major limiting factor for its use. Regular MRI monitor is mandatory. JC virus antibody should be regularly assayed for seronegative subjects.
- Alemtuzumab (annual IV infusion)
  - monoclonal antibody against CD52, leads to prolonged depletion of lymphocytes followed by lymphocyte repopulation
  - reduces relapse rate and MRI disease activity, slows down accumulation of disability, and may lead to sustained reduction of disability
  - adverse effects include infusion reactions and secondary autoimmune disorders (thyroid disease, ITP, and Goodpasture's syndrome)
  - regular monitoring of CBC, renal function, and thyroid function tests is mandatory

Symptomatic treatment

- Limb spasticity
  - baclofen (oral, intrathecal via pump in extreme patients)
  - benzodiazepines
  - dantrolene
- Neuropathic pain, trigeminal neuralgia
  - carbamazepine, oxcarbazepine
  - gabapentin, pregabalin
  - antidepressants
- Fatigue
  - amantadine, methylphenidate
- Walking impairment
  - dalfampridine

- Sexual dysfunction
  - sildenafil

Acute disseminated encephalomyelitis (ADEM)

This is an acute monophasic central demyelinating disease which manifests with varying severity. A temporal relationship (within 20 days) often exists between the onset and a febrile illness, especially a viral infection or vaccination. It is thought to be due to autoimmune mechanisms induced by viral antigens. Four varieties of ADEM may be encountered.

Post-infectious encephalomyelitis

- More common in infants and young children
- Decreased incidence with immunization
- One in 1,000 for measles virus with 25% mortality rate and major sequelae in 25–40% of survivors
- One in 10,000 for varicella-zoster virus and one in 20,000 for rubella virus; better prognosis
- Variable frequency and severity in herpes simplex virus, HIV virus, human herpes virus-6, mumps virus, influenza virus, Epstein-Barr virus, coxsackievirus type B, *Mycoplasma pneumoniae*, and *Legionella cincinnatiensis*

Post-immunization encephalomyelitis

- First reported after Pasteur developed the vaccine against rabies in 1886
- Most commonly associated with vaccination against measles (1–2 per million), mumps, and rubella

Acute haemorrhagic leucoencephalitis

- A severe form of ADEM with haemorrhagic inflammation in the white matter
- High mortality; severe morbidity in survivors

- Preceding upper respiratory tract infection common
- Differential diagnosis: viral encephalitis, brain abscess

Post-organ-transplantation encephalomyelitis

- Possibly due to long-term use of immunosuppressants resulting in secondary acute microbial infection or reactivation of latent viral infection
- May also be related to toxic effects of immunosuppressants on white matter

Pathology

The brain and spinal cord frequently appear swollen and congested. The characteristic lesions (with intense perivascular inflammatory cells and demyelination) are prominent in the white matter of the centrum ovale, cerebellum, brainstem, and spinal cord. Haemorrhage is present in severe cases. The grey matter is less affected. Neutrophils and later macrophages and lymphocytes aggregate at the lesions. Plasma proteins leak into the CSF following a breakdown of the blood-brain-barrier. The end results are astrocytic hyperplasia and gliosis.

Clinical features

The onset is often acute with fever, headache, confusion and decreased consciousness. Neck rigidity, focal neurological deficits (bilateral optic neuritis, hemiparesis, transverse myelitis, cranial nerve palsies, cerebellar ataxia) and convulsions are common. Among severe cases, death may occur within two weeks of onset. CSF analysis often shows a mild lymphocytic pleocytosis with protein elevation, and OB, IgG or myelin basic protein may be present. The differential diagnosis includes other demyelinating diseases.

Neuroimaging

- Essential for diagnosis, but lesions may not appear in the first few days.
- MRI is superior to CT.
- CT: subcortical white matter hypodensity with or without contrast enhancement
- MRI: Multiple patchy areas of increased signal in the subcortical white matter on T_2 weighted, proton density and FLAIR images (Figure 9.1b)

Treatment

- Supportive
- High-dose IV steroids to suppress a presumed aberrant immune response
- Other useful immunomodulatory therapies: plasmapheresis, IVIG

Neuromyelitis optica spectrum disorders (NMOSD)

In the original description, Devic's disease or neuromyelitis optica (NMO) was a monophasic syndrome of concurrent bilateral optic neuritis and acute transverse myelitis. In fact, most NMO patients have relapsing attacks of unilateral optic neuritis and longitudinally extensive transverse myelitis (LETM, extending over 3 or more vertebral segments). NMO-IgG are autoantibodies targeting aquaporin-4 (AQP4), a water channel protein expressed abundantly in astrocytic foot processes and ependymal cells of mammalian CNS. Since they are present in NMO but not in MS, their detection facilitates the diagnosis of NMO and other NMOSD such as recurrent myelitis without optic neuritis, and recurrent optic neuritis without myelitis, and also differentiates NMOSD from MS.

Pathology

Affected spinal cord tissue typically shows demyelination, axonal loss, grey matter involvement with necrosis, oedema, and inflammation (infiltration of lymphocytes, neutrophils, and eosinophils). The vessel walls are thickened and hyalinized. Immunohistochemistry reveals perivascular deposition of immunoglobulins and complement activation products in a rim-and-rosette pattern, and loss of aquaporin-4 from astrocytic injury and cytotoxicity. Complement activation plays a key role in the neuroinflammation in NMOSD resulting in severe astrocytic injury/loss.

Clinical features

The majority of patients present with relapsing attacks of severe optic neuritis and myelitis especially LETM. Visual blurring or loss, central scotoma, and pain on eye movements may be acute or subacute in onset. Bilateral lower limb weakness, numbness and paraesthesia, sensory loss with a sensory level, sphincter dysfunction may present acutely or subacutely. High cervical myelitis may cause life-threatening respiratory insufficiency due to intercostal and diaphragmatic weakness. Less severe short segment myelitis (extending within 2 vertebral segments) are observed in 14% of NMOSD patients. Brain involvement may present as the initial attack or relapse after previous myelitis or optic neuritis. Diverse neurological manifestations occur with brain involvement. Disabilities accumulate with permanent damage from acute attacks, which can develop after several relapses.

Treatment of acute attacks

IV pulse steroid is standard therapy. Plasmapheresis should be performed if there is no significant neurological improvement 2 weeks after pulse steroid or pulse steroid is contraindicated. IVIG can be used when pulse steroid and plasmapheresis are contraindicated.

Prophylactic treatment with immunosuppressive medications

Once the diagnosis of NMOSD is confirmed with detection of AQP4 autoantibodies, immunosuppressive medications should be initiated to prevent relapse, which can be disabling and even life-threatening. These medications include azathioprine, mycophenolate, and rituximab. Prophylactic therapeutic agents for MS are not only ineffective but also harmful for NMOSD.

CNS inflammatory demyelinating disorders with anti-myelin oligodendrocyte glycoprotein (MOG) antibody

Recently, it is recognized that about 25% of patients with clinical presentations compatible with NMOSD but no detectable AQP4 autoantibody are seropositive for anti-MOG antibody. The exact nature of this group of disorders is uncertain. Current recommendations from centres with most expertise in management of patients seropositive for anti-MOG antibody suggest oral steroid therapy for 6–12 months after treatment for acute phase (pulse steroid ± plasmapheresis or IVIG), and to consider long-term immunosuppressant therapy such as mycophenolate mofetil for relapsing cases with severe attacks.

Transverse myelitis (see Chapter 14)

Central pontine myelinolysis

This rare disorder usually complicates a severe illness or major metabolic disturbances. Associated metabolic encephalopathy (e.g., Wernicke's encephalopathy, delirium tremens) often coexists. Rapid correction of hypo- or hypernatraemia is thought to be an underlying mechanism, but this disorder may occur in chronic alcoholics or malnourished patients with normonatraemia.

Pathology

- Extensive confluent demyelination in the basal part of mid- to upper pons not conforming to any vascular territory
- Extra-pontine demyelination may also be found in the thalamus and subcortical area.
- Dense infiltration of lipid-laden macrophages; reduced number of oligodendrocytes; relative sparing of neurones

Clinical features

- Rapid deterioration in consciousness with progressive deficits over several days
- Spastic tetraparesis, conjugate gaze palsy, dysarthria, dysphagia, bulbar palsy, locked-in syndrome or coma

Investigations

- MRI brain shows hyperintense central pontine and/or extra-pontine lesions on T_2 weighted images.
- CT brain not sensitive
- Normal CSF

Treatment

- Prevention is most important.
- Treat underlying condition, e.g., IV thiamine for Wernicke's encephalopathy.
- Avoid rapid correction of hypo- or hypernatraemia, the recommended rate being 0.5–1 mmol/l/hr.
- Supportive treatment for established condition

Prognosis

- Poor
- High mortality and morbidity

10 Autoimmune Disorders of the Nervous System

Autoimmune neurological disorders are increasingly recognized through identifying novel antibodies which target different membrane and cytosolic autoantigens in neurons, glia cells, peripheral nerves, neuromuscular junction, and muscle. Neurological manifestations are diverse, depending on the anatomical site of involvement. Detection of the specific autoantibodies assists in the diagnosis of these disorders and their differentiation from diseases sharing similar clinical features. It is important to consider autoimmune neurological disorders since they are potentially treatable and some are associated with malignancy (paraneoplastic).

SELECTED ENTITIES

Autoimmune encephalitis

Autoimmune encephalitis has been increasingly recognized in recent years as a potentially treatable cause of encephalopathies, behavioural abnormalities, cognitive impairment, epilepsy, and sleep disturbance. Diagnosis is facilitated by detection of characteristic autoantibodies targeting neuronal intracellular or surface (membrane or synaptic) antigens in the serum and/or CSF of patients. In general, patients with autoantibodies against neuronal intracellular antigens have limited response to immunotherapy, whereas those with autoantibodies against surface antigens have good response to immunotherapy. Patients of all ages are affected and underlying neoplasms are detected in some of them, consistent with a paraneoplastic nature. It is particularly important to be aware that psychiatric symptoms are common in some patients and may be initial presenting features. In most cases, CSF lymphocytic pleocytosis is present with normal CSF glucose and normal or mildly elevated CSF protein levels. MRI brain is particularly useful in limbic encephalitis as most patients with autoimmune limbic encephalitis have uni- or bilateral T2/FLAIR hyperintense signal in medial temporal lobes. It is important to suspect autoimmune encephalitis in patients with rapidly progressive encephalopathy of uncertain aetiology, especially in the presence of (1) multifocal symptoms with or without MRI abnormalities, and (2) CSF lymphocytic pleocytosis.

A common form of autoimmune encephalitis associated with antibodies targeting neuronal surface auto-antigens is anti-NMDA receptor (anti-NMDAR) encephalitis, characterized by the detection of autoantibodies against the GluN1 subunit of the NMDAR. Other antibodies targeting neuronal surface auto-antigens were subsequently identified in patients with encephalitis who improved with immunotherapy. These include antibodies targeting the following auto-antigens:

- Leucine-rich glioma inactivated-1 (LGI-1)
- Contactin-associated protein-like 2 (Caspr2)
- AMPA receptor (AMPAR)
- GABAa receptor (GABAaR)
- GABAb receptor (GABAbR)
- Glycine receptor (GlyR)
- Dopamine receptor (DR2)

Anti-NMDAR encephalitis

Clinical features

All ages are affected, but usually in young adults and children (median age 21 years), women are affected more (~80%). About 38% of all patients (46% of all women) had an underlying neoplasm, most common in patients between 12 and 45 years of age; 94% of tumours were ovarian teratoma, 2% extraovarian teratomas, and 4% other tumours.

About 70% patients develop prodromal symptoms of headache, nausea, vomiting, and fever. This is followed by acute onset of behavioural abnormalities such as confusion, agitation, aggression, anxiety, insomnia, paranoia, delusions, hallucinations, mania, psychosis, sexual disinhibition, and catatonia. Many patients are treated as viral encephalitis initially, and presentation to psychiatrists is common. Dyskinesia including oro-facial dyskinesia, choreoathetosis, ballismus, and rigidity then develops, followed by impairment of consciousness which can progress to coma. Autonomic dysfunction is common and manifests as labile blood pressure, tachycardia, hypersalivation, hyperthermia, central hypoventilation, bradycardia, and even cardiac pauses. Seizures are typically generalized and complex partial, and status epilepticus can occur at any stage. MRI brain is normal in about two-thirds of patients; in the remaining one-third, the abnormal features include non-specific cortical or subcortical T2W signals (especially in the medial temporal and infratentorial regions) and demyelinating lesions.

It is important to have a high index of suspicion of anti-NMDAR encephalitis in patients presenting with protracted clinical course of complexed neurological and psychiatric manifestations. Prompt assay of CSF for anti-NMDAR antibody facilitates the diagnosis, as many patients are seronegative for the antibody.

Pathogenetic mechanism

Anti-NMDAR antibody is pathogenic by binding to the NMDAR on neuronal/synaptic membrane. This leads to internalization of the receptors, reducing the number and density of NMDAR, and impairing synaptic function.

Treatment

- Meticulous supportive care with close monitoring
- Anti-epileptic drugs and assisted ventilation for patients with severe impairment of consciousness and status epilepticus
- IV pulse steroid, IVIG and plasmapheresis as first-line therapies
- Second-line agents are used when first-line therapy fails. Examples are rituximab (anti-CD20 monoclonal antibody) and combination of cyclophosphamide and rituximab.
- Prompt tumour ablative therapy for underlying tumour

- Immunosuppressant therapy for 12 months recommended for patients without underlying tumour to prevent relapse
- Reassessment for recurrent or contralateral teratoma for non-responders or for relapse

Prognosis

- Mortality rate ~7%, mostly during acute stage
- Good clinical outcome (modified Rankin scale score 0–2) ~80% at 24 months
- Relapse occurs in 12–20% of patients.
- In general, young women with ovarian teratoma have better prognosis than patients with no underlying tumour found.

Limbic encephalitis associated with LGI1 antibodies

Initially, antibodies against voltage-gated potassium channel (VGKC) were reported to be detected in the sera of some patients with limbic encephalitis. It was subsequently clarified that in the majority of these patients, the autoantibodies in fact bind specifically to LGI1, a protein involved in a trans-synaptic complex that includes VGKC. Limbic encephalitis associated with LGI1 antibodies typically affects middle-aged or elderly patients, male more than female (2:1), who present with marked impairment of short-term memory, confusion, and frequent seizures. Hyponatremia develops in 60% of patients. Some have myoclonic-like jerks in the face, arm or leg (facio-brachial dystonic seizure) preceding onset of encephalitis. Recognition of this seizure and early diagnosis by detection of LGI1 antibodies are important as early treatment of these seizures with immunotherapy may prevent development of encephalitis and cognitive impairment. Some patients with LGI1 antibodies develop confusion and cognitive impairment rapidly over a few months suggestive of rapidly progressive dementia, mimicking CJD.

Underlying thymoma is found in less than 10% of patients. There are no guidelines on treatment of limbic encephalitis associated with LGI1 antibodies. IVIG, corticosteroids, and plasmapheresis are currently used, which usually result in clinical improvement.

Autoimmune encephalitis associated with antibodies against neuronal intracellular antigens

Multifocal involvement is present. Neurological manifestations are therefore diverse, including subacute onset of progressive encephalomyelitis, brainstem encephalitis, focal cortical encephalitis, limbic encephalitis, diencephalitic encephalitis, and cerebellar degeneration. The majority (96–98%) have underlying malignancy, such as small cell carcinoma, thymoma, Ca breast, ovary, and testis. Detection of associated autoantibodies including anti-Hu (ANNA-1), anti-CRMP5, anti-amphiphysin, anti-Ri (ANNA-2), anti-Yo (PCA-1), and anti-Ma2 aids diagnosis. Treatment of underlying tumour is the most important measure as there is limited response to immunotherapy.

Stiff-person syndrome (SPS)

SPS is characterized by muscle rigidity and spasm predominantly affecting axial, low back, and proximal limb muscles, which occur spontaneously or are triggered by stimuli such as auditory, visual, tactile, and emotional upset. Sustained contraction of antagonist groups of muscles leads to restricted range of movement, slow motion, muscle hypertrophy, and abnormal postures with characteristic hyperlordosis, and in severe cases, marked truncal rigidity with gait impairment, imbalance, frequent falls, and hypo- or immobility. Some experience chronic muscle pain. The mechanism is related to dysfunction of the inhibitory GABAergic system. EMG of affected muscles reveals continuous motor unit activity. Most patients have high serum titres of glutamic acid decarboxylase (GAD65) antibodies without underlying tumour, and can develop coexisting cerebellar ataxia associated with diabetes and thyroid dysfunction. About 5% of SPS patients have underlying breast cancer or small cell lung carcinoma, usually associated with anti-amphiphysin antibodies instead of GAD65 antibodies. Both the symptoms and EMG improve with GABA agonists such as diazepam and oral baclofen. Other symptomatic therapies that may be effective include levetiracetam, botulinum toxin, intravenous or subcutaneous opiates, and intrathecal baclofen. Immunotherapy should be considered in most SPS patients. IVIG improves muscle spasms, mobility, frequency of falls, and ADL. Plasmapheresis and rituximab have been used with variable success.

Acute inflammatory demyelinating polyneuroradiculopathy (Guillain-Barrè syndrome) (see Chapter 15)

Chronic inflammatory demyelinating polyneuroradiculopathy (see Chapter 15)

Myasthenia gravis (MG)

MG is a neuromuscular junction disorder characterized by weakness and fatigability of skeletal muscles. Its prevalence and incidence are similar in different populations, being 43–64 per million and 2–6 per million respectively.

Classification

Adult MG (onset after puberty)

I.   Ocular disease (restricted ocular involvement more than 2 years after onset)
IIA. Mild generalized disease
IIB. Moderately severe generalized disease
III. Fulminating disease
IV.   Late severe disease: marked increase in severity after 2 or more years of mild disease

Paediatric MG (onset before puberty)

I.   Transient neonatal MG: born to MG mother, onset 24 hours to first few days after birth
IIA. Early onset juvenile MG (congenital MG): presenting before 2 years old
IIB. Late onset juvenile MG: resembles adult disease

III. Familial infantile MG: rare; onset at birth, remitting course, spares external ocular muscles, unaffected mother and affected siblings

IV. Familial limb girdle MG: rare; only limb girdle weakness

D-penicillamine induced MG

MG following therapeutic use of D-penicillamine

Pathophysiology and pathogenesis

In MG, auto-antibodies targeting the acetylcholine receptors (AChRs) reduce the availability of receptors by degrading them at a faster rate, occupying the active site of the receptors, and damaging the post-synaptic membrane via complement activation. In addition, the post-synaptic folds are flattened. These factors account for the small end-plate potentials which fail to trigger muscle action potentials.

Thymus abnormalities are common in MG patients and include hyperplasia, invasive or non-invasive thymomas. The role of thymus in MG is unclear. The myoid cells within the thymus, which bear AChRs on their surface, may serve as a source of auto-antigens and trigger the autoimmune reaction within the thymus.

Genetic factors probably play a role in determining the susceptibility to MG. HLA profiles are different in MG patients of different races and appear to be associated with variants of MG. In Caucasians, A1, B8, and DR3 are more common. In Japanese, B5 and B12 are more common. In Chinese, BW46 and DR9 are associated with juvenile onset, and ocular MG with low anti-AChR titres. Family members of patients with MG are much more likely to develop MG when compared with the general population.

Clinical picture

MG is more common in females. The disease may present at any age, but more commonly in the first three decades. Any muscle group (ocular, bulbar, trunk, limb, respiratory) may be involved, either singly or more often in various combinations. Fatigability of the involved muscles is a characteristic feature. In the course of disease, ocular presentation may evolve to generalized MG. MG is often associated with other autoimmune diseases, especially thyroid disorders. Other associated diseases include thymoma (in about 15% of generalized MG patients), non-thymic neoplasms, and DM.

Diagnosis

Look for specific features of the muscle weakness, namely, variability and fatigability. There is also a predilection for eye muscles, which gives rise to partial ptosis and/or diplopia.

The Edrophonium (Tensilon) test

Dramatic improvement of ptosis, dysconjugate gaze or nasal speech following IV edrophonium is diagnostic of MG. However, a brief response may not be noticeable to a casual examiner, and improvement in limb muscle power should be interpreted with care. False positive test may occur in MND and inflammatory myopathies. A double-blind Tensilon test enhances the objectivity of the test.

Anti-AChR anti-bodies (Anti-AChR)

The titre is raised in most patients with generalized MG, but may be undetected especially ocular MG. The correlation between anti-AChR titres and clinical severity is poor. For high-quality assay, false positive results may occur in primary biliary cirrhosis and graft-versus-host disease. Generalized MG patients seronegative for anti-AChR may be seropositive for anti-muscle-specific kinase antibodies (anti-MuSK). MG patients with anti-MuSK in general are more likely to have frequent MG crises, severe oculobulbar involvement, and facial lingual atrophy.

Clinical neurophysiology

• Repetitive nerve stimulation. Sensitivity is around 80% if the proximal and distal muscles are tested. Significant decrement is defined as follows: the amplitude of the fourth or fifth cMAP to a train of low frequency nerve stimuli falls by 10% or more of the first cMAP (Table 10.1).

Table 10.1   Repetitive nerve stimulation in neuromuscular disorders

NMJ defect	Disorder	cMAP	Slow RNS	Fast RNS
Postsynaptic	Myasthenia gravis	Normal	Decrement	Normal or decrement
Presynaptic	Eaton-Lambert syndrome	Low	Decrement	increment

cMAP = compound muscle action potential; NMJ = neuromuscular junction
RNS = repetitive nerve stimulation

• Concentric needle EMG. It serves to exclude other diseases which mimic MG, e.g., myositis or thyroid myopathy.
• Single fibre EMG. It is a highly sensitive but not a specific test of neuromuscular transmission. Increased jittering and/or intermittent block are found in the MAPs.

Other investigations

• CK: to exclude muscle disease
• Thyroid function tests: dysthyroid eye disease, concomitant thyroid disease
• Auto-antibodies: anti-striated muscle antibodies, anti-thyroid antibodies, antinuclear factor, rheumatoid factor
• CT/MRI thorax: thymic enlargement due to hyperplasia or tumour

Differential diagnosis

Dysthyroid eye disease

It is characterized by exophthalmos, fixed inferior rectus, distortion of visual axis, negative Tensilon test, and thickening of extraocular muscles on CT or MR orbit. Patients with MG may have coexisting dysthyroid eye disease.

Myopathies (see also Chapter 16)

- Congenital: Presents at birth or early in life with normal bulbar muscles and negative Tensilon test
- Metabolic: Usually progressive proximal muscle weakness
- Endocrine: thyrotoxicosis, hypothyroidism, Cushing's syndrome
- Mitochondrial encephalomyopathy: e.g., retinal degeneration, heart block, encephalopathy
- Polymyositis and dermatomyositis (see Chapter 16)
- Myasthenia syndrome – Eaton-Lambert syndrome (*vide infra*)

Treatment

Treatment should be individualized. Age, severity of disease, and degree of functional impairment are factors to be considered. Most patients improve with treatment. In general, the treatment strategy is as follows.

Ocular MG
- Anti-cholinesterase, steroids ± azathioprine
- Response to treatment not as good as generalized MG

Generalized MG
- Mild cases: anti-cholinesterase
- Moderate to severe cases without radiological evidence of thymoma: anti-cholinesterase, thymectomy, steroid, azathioprine/mycophenolate

Thymoma
- Thymectomy obligatory in all forms of MG
- Post-operative irradiation or chemotherapy for invasive thymoma

Anti-cholinesterase

It produces dramatic improvement in some patients. Pyridostigmine (Mestinon) is most commonly used because it has fewer gastrointestinal side effects. It retards the enzymatic hydrolysis of ACh at the cholinergic synapse, and may have direct agonist effects. Begin with a small dose and gradually increase to the optimum dose. The dosage is adjusted according to clinical response. Different muscle groups have different responses to the same dose of Mestinon. Hence, underdose for one group and overdose for another group of muscles may occur at the same time.

The side effects consist of:
- Muscarinic effects include nausea, vomiting, abdominal cramps and diarrhoea, increased bronchial and pharyngeal secretions. Anticholinergic drugs (e.g., atropine or probanthine) ameliorate these side effects.
- Nicotinic effect: cholinergic weakness

Thymectomy

The indications are suspected thymoma, generalized MG of moderate or severe grade, and possibly disabling ocular MG. Outcome is satisfactory in 50–70% of patients. Good prognostic factors are the female gender, age younger than 45 years and early disease, whereas poor prognostic factors are age over 45 and presence of thymoma. Improvement usually occurs in 6–12 months after surgery, but delayed remission after 2 years is possible. Post-operative irradiation with or without chemotherapy is indicated in invasive thymoma.

Corticosteroids

Steroid therapy is effective in 80% patients with MG. The recommended regime is to begin with a small dose of prednisolone and to increase gradually until improvement is observed. When patient has been stabilized for a period of time, the dosage may be reduced, particularly if the patient is also on azathioprine.

Immunosuppressive drugs

Azathioprine is effective in most patients with MG, but its effect is delayed by 4–6 months. It may be used as a steroid-sparing drug or in combination with steroids in resistant cases. Mycophenolate mofetil (MMF) probably has similar efficacy but fewer side effects.

Cyclosporine is an alternative. Although its side effects in general are more serious, it is safe for pregnant women. Rituximab is increasingly used in patients refractory to conventional immunosuppressants (steroid and azathioprine or MMF or cyclosporine). Cyclophosphamide may be useful in refractory cases, but severe toxicity is a major concern.

Plasmapheresis and IVIG

Virtually all patients with MG improve at least temporarily following plasmapheresis. The onset of action is usually within 48 hours after the first exchange. Its beneficial effect is short-lived but may last for weeks or months. Concomitant immunosuppression is often necessary. A course usually consists of 4–6 exchanges (alternate days or once every 3 days). More frequent exchanges are not associated with greater benefits.

The major indications are myasthenic crisis and pre-operative preparation for thymectomy or other surgical procedures. However, it may be used for initiating improvement that may be sustained by other forms of immunotherapy, and for patients who fail to respond to other forms of treatment.

An alternative is IVIG. The onset of action is within 1 week and duration of response lasts 4–8 weeks. The mechanism may be due to down-regulation of anti-AChR. Hypersensitivity reaction may occur and the cost of treatment is comparable to plasma exchange.

Crisis in MG

Crisis in myasthenia is a neurological emergency. It is defined as deterioration in neuromuscular function within days, with severe respiratory and bulbar involvement. Respiratory assistance is often required. It can be classified into three types: myasthenic, cholinergic, and mixed (Table 10.2).

Table 10.2   Crisis in MG

Myasthenic crisis	Cholinergic crisis
Respiratory failure	Abdominal cramps
Poor cough and swallowing effort	Nausea, vomiting, diarrhoea
Generalized muscle weakness	Weakness ± fasciculations
Improved by Tensilon	Worsened by Tensilon

Note: Tensilon test is not helpful in differentiating myasthenic from cholinergic crisis, and it may cause further deterioration. If doubt exists, cholinesterase inhibitor should be discontinued temporarily to exclude cholinergic crisis.

Management

Manage the patient in the ICU, since intubation and mechanical ventilation are often required and patients may have unstable haemodynamics. Nasogastric tube feeding is necessary to prevent aspiration.

The indications for respiratory support are dyspnoea, forced vital capacity less than 1 litre, oxygen desaturation, hypercapnia or acidosis.

Treat/pre-empt precipitating factors:
• Infections especially aspiration pneumonia
• Prophylactic plasma exchange in severe or labile cases before thymectomy
• Avoid the following drugs which are known to induce deterioration in neuromuscular function:
    – Aminoglycosides
    – D-penicillamine (absolutely contraindicated)

- All neuromuscular blockers
- Local anaesthetics, e.g., lignocaine
- Sedatives
- Anti-arrhythmics, e.g., quinine, quinidine, procainamide
- ß-blockers, e.g., propanolol, timolol eyedrops
- Calcium channel blockers
- Avoid rapid withdrawal of steroids
- Treat any coexisting hyperthyroidism

Plasmapheresis or IVIG is often required to hasten recovery of neuromuscular function. Anti-cholinesterase should be stopped for a few days and then reintroduced at low dose and titrated according to clinical response. Long-term immunosuppressive therapy should be considered.

Special situations

Anaesthetic management of the MG patient

Local or spinal anaesthesia is preferred to inhalational anaesthesia. Neuromuscular blockers should be avoided if possible. MG patients usually require assisted ventilation for a longer time after surgery. Ensure adequate respiratory function before assisted ventilation is discontinued.

MG in pregnancy

The myasthenic status may be worse, better or unchanged during pregnancy. If deterioration occurs, it is usually in the third trimester or postpartum period for multipara or during the first trimester for primigravida. However, therapeutic abortion is not indicated. Cytotoxic drugs and IV anti-cholinesterase should not be used.

Labour and delivery are usually normal. Regional anaesthesia is preferred for delivery or caesarean section. Plasmapheresis is a safe procedure in case of deterioration.

Look out for neonatal MG in the baby. Breast-feeding is generally safe.

Myasthenic syndrome (Eaton-Lambert syndrome)

It is due to a pre-synaptic defect with impaired release of ace-tycholine. The pathogenesis involves auto-antibodies (detected in about 50% of patients) directed against voltage-gated calcium channels at cholinergic nerve terminals. It is associated with malignancies (e.g., carcinoma of bronchus) and immunological disorders. It affects proximal and truncal muscles, and occasion-ally ocular and bulbar muscles. Other symptoms (e.g., myalgia, muscle stiffness, paraesthesia, dry mouth, and impotence) may be present. A characteristic feature is diminished reflexes, which are enhanced after exertion; this is the clinical equivalent of the phenomenon of marked increase of the small cMAP with tetanic stimulation. Potentiation may be seen following repetitive nerve stimulation. Tensilon test is negative. Specific treatment consists of 3,4-diaminopyridine, pyridostigmine, immunosuppression and successful treatment of underlying malignancy.

Polymyositis and Dermatomyositis (see Chapter 16)

11 Dementia

Dementia is a clinical syndrome of impaired cognitive function in multiple domains but with preserved consciousness. Cognitive impairment involves deterioration of memory, intellect, concentration, comprehension, executive functions, and specific cortical functions (aphasia, apraxia, agnosia, acalculia, visuo-spatial disturbance). Other features, e.g., abnormal movements, seizures, pyramidal and extrapyramidal signs, cerebellar ataxia, gait disturbance, and primitive reflexes, may also be present.

Causes

A large number of neurological diseases can cause dementia (Table 11.1), but most of them are uncommon. By far the most common cause of dementia is Alzheimer's disease (AD), followed by vascular dementia.

Table 11.1   Causes of dementia

Causes	
Neurodegeneration	AD, Pick's disease, Huntington's disease, diffuse Lewy body disease, Parkinson's disease, multisystem atrophy, progressive supranuclear palsy, spinocerebellar degeneration, CBGD, cerebral gliosis and related conditions, progressive myoclonic epilepsies
Vascular dementia	Multiple lacunes, cortical or subcortical infarct/ischaemia
Infection/transmissible disease	Syphilis, cerebral AIDS, PML, SSPE, progressive rubella panencephalitis, transmissible prion diseases

Table 11.1   (continued)

Causes	
Tumour/altered intracranial pressure	Intracerebral tumour, e.g., glioma involving corpus callosum Extracerebral mass: frontal meningioma, chronic subdural haematoma Normal pressure hydrocephalus
Post-irradiation damage	
Toxic substance	Chronic alcohol consumption, heavy metals (e.g., lead, mercury, manganese, aluminium), organic chemicals (e.g., carbon tetrachloride)
Metabolic disorder	Chronic hepatic encephalopathy, hypo- or hyperthyroidism, hypo- or hypercalcaemia, hypopituitarism, porphyria, Wilson's disease, gangliosidoses, cerebro-tendinous xanthomatosis
Blood disorder	Polycythaemia rubra vera, hyperviscosity syndrome, chronic severe anaemia
Other conditions	Vitamin B_1 or B_{12} deficiency, Whipple's disease, multiple sclerosis

Diagnosis

History

It is important to obtain a comprehensive history which includes details of the symptoms, past health, drug and family history, recent life events and (e.g., bereavement, retirement, loss of employment). Specific problems in daily living and employment should be explored. Depressive symptoms (e.g., early morning wakening, lethargy) should be looked for. It is also vital to get a history from close relatives or independent carers.

Examination

A general physical examination and a full neurological examination should be performed. Higher mental functions should be assessed for the domain and severity of the deficits:

Memory   – immediate recall
            – short-term memory (new recent information)
            – long-term memory (past personal and public events)
Language   – word finding, word errors
            – comprehension
            – reading and writing abilities
Visuo-spatial orientation   – dressing skills, apraxia, agnosia
Mathematical skills   – handling money, shopping
Problem-solving ability   – concrete thinking
Personal and social conduct   – paranoia, disinhibition, symp-
                                 toms of depression, delusions and
                                 hallucinations

The Mini-Mental State Examination (MMSE) is a good screening test (Table 11.2).

Differential diagnosis

Certain conditions may be misdiagnosed as dementia:
- Primary psychiatric disorders, which are presented as pseu-dodementia, account for about 10% of presumed dementia. Depression is the most common form. Schizophrenia, especially if associated with depressive symptoms, can be misdiagnosed as dementia. In these cases, patients are often able to describe their symptoms in detail.
- Oligophrenia (longstanding poverty of intellect)
- Isolated disorder of higher cerebral function, e.g., dysphasia, visual agnosia
- Delirium is an acute confusional state with fluctuating con-sciousness which can be precipitated by alcohol, drugs (e.g., anticholinergics), systemic diseases (e.g., heart or lung diseases, urinary tract infection), metabolic disorders (e.g., uraemia or hepatic encephalopathy), or acute neurological events (e.g., stroke, trauma).

Table 11.2 Mini-Mental State Examination (MMSE)

Domain tested	Score
Orientation	
Year, month, date, day, time	_____ /5
Country, town, district, hospital, ward	_____ /5
Registration	
Examiner names three items (e.g., apple, table, penny).	
Patient asked to repeat the three items—score one for each correct answer.	
Then patient to learn three names (i.e., repeat until correct).	_____ /3
Attention and calculation	
Subtract 7 from 100, then repeat from result, etc. Stop after 65. 100, 93, 86, 79, 72, 65. (Alternative: recall '27984' backwards)	_____ /5
Recall	
Ask for three objects learnt earlier.	_____ /3
Language	
Name a pencil and watch.	_____ /2
Repeat 'No ifs, ands, or buts'.	_____ /1
Give a 3-stage command. Score one for each stage (e.g., 'Raise your left hand, place your right index finger on your nose, and then on your left ear.')	_____ /3
Ask patient to read and obey a written command on a piece of paper stating: 'Close your eyes.'	_____ /1
Ask patient to write a sentence. Score if it is sensible and has a subject and a verb.	_____ /1
Copying	
Ask patient to copy a pair of intersecting pentagons.	_____ /1

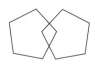

Adapted from Wade D. *Measurement in Neurological Rehabilitation* (Oxford: Oxford University Press, 1992), 133–134.

Investigations

Investigations (Table 11.3) should be performed to exclude potentially reversible causes of dementia.

Table 11.3   Investigations of dementia

Investigations	To detect
CBC	Anaemia, polycythaemia, macrocytosis
Vasculitic screen, ESR	Vasculitis
LFT, RFT	Metabolic encephalopathy
VDRL, FTA-Abs	Neurosyphilis
TSH	Hypo- or hyperthyroidism
Serum B_{12} and folate	B_{12} or folate deficiency
CSF studies	Chronic meningitis or neurosyphilis
EEG	Periodic complexes suggest CJD; triphasic waves indicate metabolic encephalopathy
ECG	Arrhythmias, ischaemic heart disease
CXR	Cardiomegaly
CT/MRI brain	Pattern of cerebral atrophies, infarcts, hydrocephalus, other focal lesions, e.g., subdural haematoma, tumour
Copper studies and slit-lamp examination	Wilson's disease

Management

Treat reversible causes, e.g., hydrocephalus, hypo- or hyperthyroidism, cerebral vasculitis, neurosyphilis, vitamin B_{12} deficiency. Pseudodementia from depression responds to antidepressants.

However, there is at present no curative treatment for most cases of dementia. Supportive management should be made available to the patient and the carers. These include discussion with the patient's family, referral to patient support groups, and liaison with psychiatrist and social worker. More advanced cases may benefit from day-care centres and long-term institutional care. Symptomatic control may be required. The judicious use of

neuroleptic drugs for confusion, aggressive behaviour, and paranoia is indicated in certain patients.

Doctors may be asked to certify the mental capacity of patients
under their care. Mental capacity is task-specific. Whether a patient
has the requisite capacity for the task, e.g., to execute a legal document, depends on two factors, viz. the degree of cognitive dysfunction and complexity of the task. A thorough assessment of these
two factors is mandatory and the findings must be documented
in detail.

SELECTED ENTITIES

Mild cognitive impairment (MCI)

Healthy aging is associated with minimal, if any, cognitive impairment. However, subtle cognitive impairment, known as age-asso-
ciated cognitive impairment, is likely to be present in the elderly
with co-morbidities such as stroke, diabetes, hypertension, heart
failure. MCI describes a condition with memory impairment
greater than would be expected for age but otherwise preserved
general cognitive function. Synonyms of MCI include dementia
prodrome, incipient dementia, and isolated memory impairment.

MCI is diagnosed using the following criteria:
1. Memory complaint corroborated by an informant
2. Normal general cognitive function
3. Normal activities of daily living
4. Memory impairment adjusted for age and education
5. Lack of sufficient evidence of dementia

MCI is a transitional state between normal cognition and early
AD with a conversion rate to AD at 10–15% per year compared to
1–2% per year for the normal elderly.

MCI is a heterogeneous condition and at least three subtypes
are recognized.
1. Amnesic MCI: typical form with predominant memory impairment and an annual conversion rate to AD at 10–15%

2. Multiple domain MCI: mild cognitive impairment in more than one cognitive domain but inadequate to constitute dementia
3. Single non-memory domain MCI: impairment in a single domain other than memory e.g., language function or executive function

Treatment of MCI is not well-defined.

Alzheimer's disease

It is the most common cause of dementia (50–70% of all cases). The prevalence is about 2% in the age group of 65–69 years, but rises to 20% in those more than 80 years of age. Although most cases are sporadic, autosomal dominant familial cases exist. Concomitant cerebrovascular disease is not uncommon and may contribute to cognitive decline (mixed dementia).

Neuropathology

Cortical argyrophilic plaques are degenerating axons and synaptic structures clustered around a core of amyloid protein which is derived from a larger amyloid precursor protein. Neurofibrillary tangles are paired helical filamentous material derived from the microtubule-associated protein tau. Both plaques and tangles are characteristic pathological findings, and the temporal lobes are usually most afflicted.

Clinical features

- Insidious onset
- Memory loss especially recent memory (encoding deficits and impaired recognition)
- Parietal symptoms, e.g., dyspraxia, dysphasia, agnosia
- Visuo-spatial disorientation
- Language impairment (word finding and comprehension)
- Mood changes, e.g., agitation, restlessness
- Change in personality, e.g., lack of spontaneity, apathy, paranoia

- Frank psychotic symptoms, e.g., delusions and hallucinations
- At the terminal stage, the patient is bed-bound and incontinent. Other neurological deficits, e.g., pyramidal and extrapyramidal features, may also be present.

Diagnosis

Specific potentially reversible causes of dementia should be excluded. Routine blood and CSF examinations are normal. CT brain frequently shows cortical atrophy, but MRI brain may show more specific focal atrophy in the hippocampi and temporal lobes. EEG shows early diffuse slowing. Fluorodeoxyglucose ([^{18}F] FDG) PET imaging shows widespread metabolic deficits in the neocortical association areas (in the parietotemporal, medial temporal, entorhinal cortex and hippocampus), sparing the basal ganglia, cerebellum, and visual cortex has been shown in Alzheimer's dementia but it is not in routine clinical use.

The diagnostic categories include:
- Definite Alzheimer's dementia – diagnosis at post-mortem
- Probable Alzheimer's dementia – typical clinical features without histological confirmation
- Possible Alzheimer's dementia – atypical clinical features

Treatment

Acetylcholinesterase inhibitors: They inhibit degradation of ACh within synapses. Donepezil (Aricept), rivastigmine (Exelon) or galantamine (Reminyl) is indicated in early to moderately advanced AD. The common side effects include anorexia, nausea, vomiting, diarrhoea, and weight loss. In general, they can delay the deterioration for about 18 months.

NMDA antagonist: Memantine (Ebixa), a non-competitive NMDA-receptor blocker, prevents excessive NMDA activation without interruption of normal NMDA transmission. Combined use with a cholinesterase inhibitor may have a synergistic action. Side effects are minimal.

Behavioural strategies: Provide emotional support; emphasize pleasant events; adhere to daily routines

Antipsychotics and anxiolytics:
Conventional antipsychotics – haloperidol, chlorpromazine, thioridazine
Atypical neuroleptics – quetiapine, risperidone, olanzapine
Mood stabilizer – carbamazepine, valproate

Prognosis

There is progressive deterioration and the median survival from diagnosis is between 7 and 10 years.

Vascular dementia

It accounts for about 15% of all dementia. The risk factors are those for CVD and include hypertension, stroke, ischaemic heart disease and peripheral vascular disease. It is therefore important to identify and treat these risk factors if present.

CVD may result in dementia via one or more of the following mechanisms:
1. A single large infarct
2. A small strategic infarct, e.g., thalamus
3. Multiple large infarcts
4. Subcortical arteriosclerotic encephalopathy (Binswanger's disease)
5. A single vascular insult on top of preclinical dementia

Clinical features

- Cumulative episodic events with stepwise deterioration
- Memory for recent events is affected first.
- Somatic symptoms, e.g., dizziness
- Nocturnal confusion
- Relative preservation of personality
- Retention of insight until advanced stage

- Gait dyspraxia
- Pyramidal signs
- Pseudobulbar palsy
- Primitive reflexes
- Hypertension, retinopathy, cardiomegaly

Management

Galantamine, rivastigmine, donepezil, and memantine can improve cognitive function in patients with vascular dementia. Modification of vascular risk factors is essential in reducing the incidence of vascular dementia.

Prognosis

The clinical course may be static or progressive. Death tends to be associated with strokes or cardiac events.

Fronto-temporal dementia (FTD)

FTD is a group of dementia (which includes primary progressive aphasia and behavioural-variant FTD) characterized by prominent abnormal behavioural features, language, and executive dysfunction. It has a younger age of onset, typically less than 65 years. Although the majority of cases are sporadic, some cases have been linked to mutations in several genes. Some patients may develop features of other neurodegenerative disorders in more advanced stages of the disease, such as the pyramidal signs and parkinsonian features. MRI brain shows atrophy predominantly of the frontal and temporal lobes and frontoinsular region. The diagnosis may be difficult initially as it can mimic various psychiatric disorders because of prominent abnormal behaviours such as obsessive-compulsiveness, apathy, depression, delusion, and euphoria. These behavioural symptoms can be ameliorated by atypical neuroleptics and antidepressants. Cholinesterase inhibitors and memantine are not helpful in FTD. The prognosis is poor with death usually occurring about 8 years after symptom onset.

Prion diseases (spongiform encephalopathies)

There are several types of prion diseases and the common features include: disease process confined to CNS, prolonged incubation period, progressive clinical course, reactive astrocytosis, and vacuolation of affected neurons. These diseases are caused by transmissible prion particles. Prions are small proteinaceous infectious particles devoid of nucleic acids which resist inactivation by routine procedures.

Creutzfeldt-Jakob disease (CJD)

CJD is a progressive spongiform encephalopathy resulting in dementia, myoclonus, extrapyramidal and pyramidal signs. Its neuropathology typically consists of vacuolation and loss of neurons with hypertrophy and proliferation of glial cells, mostly in the cerebral cortex. Transmission has been implicated from corneal grafts, pituitary growth hormone, and contaminated neurosurgical instruments. Familial CJD consists of about 10% of cases. Death usually occurs within a year. In CJD, EEG shows typical periodic high-voltage, polyspike or triphasic sharp wave complexes (1–2 Hz) with suppressed background activity. MRI brain (DWI and FLAIR sequences) which show abnormal hyperintensity in cortical gyri ("cortical ribboning") is useful to help diagnose CJD.

Variant CJD (vCJD) is causally linked to bovine spongiform encephalopathy. Its clinical features include a younger age of onset, early psychiatric manifestations (most often depression) and painful sensory symptoms followed by rapidly progressive dementia, ataxia, and finally akinetic mutism. Its pathology is characterized by florid plaques with dense prion protein deposits on immunohistochemical staining. MRI brain shows high signal intensity within the posterior thalamus (pulvinar nucleus), the so-called 'pulvinar' sign. Tonsillar biopsy is helpful for diagnosis.

Precautions in suspected CJD cases:
- Correct disposal of used EEG electrodes and lumbar puncture needles
- Sterilization of contaminated instruments with 2M NaOH and autoclaving at >120°C for 4.5 hours

Normal pressure hydrocephalus (see Chapter 5)

12 Impaired Consciousness and Brain Death

Impaired consciousness

Consciousness refers to a state of awareness of self and the surrounding, and coma is a serious impairment of consciousness. Wakefulness requires a functioning brainstem, and awareness of self and environment requires a functioning cerebral cortex.

Loss of consciousness implies loss of awareness and responsiveness. There is a four-point continuum of arousal:

- Alert: normal state of arousal
- Lethargy: lies between alert and stupor
- Stupor: unresponsive and only aroused by vigorous and repeated stimuli
- Coma: unarousable unresponsiveness

Delirium refers to altered consciousness with reduced attention to environmental stimuli and is diagnosed by at least two of the following features: perceptual disturbance, incoherent speech, disturbed sleep-wake cycle, and altered psychomotor activity.

Glasgow Coma Scale (GCS)

The GCS (Table 12.1) provides a means to assess the severity of impaired consciousness and a baseline to judge improvement or deterioration.

Table 12.1   Glasgow Coma Scale (GCS)

Best motor response		Best verbal response		Eye opening	
Obeys	M6	Oriented	V5	Spontaneous	E4
Localizes*	5	Confused conversation	4	To speech	3
Withdraws*	4	Inappropriate words	3	To pain	2
Abnormal flexion*	3	Incomprehensible sounds	2	Nil	1
Extensor response*	2	Nil	1		
Nil*	1				

*to painful stimuli
Range of scores: 3–15; Coma: 3–6; Stupor: 7–10; Lethargy: 11–14

Aetiology

Clinical differentiation between CNS and non-CNS causes is important (Table 12.2).

- CVD: cortical infarct, ICH, SAH, hypertensive encephalopathy
- Intoxication or drug overdose: alcohol, major or minor tranquilizers, opiates, carbon monoxide
- Trauma: subdural or epidural haematoma, brain contusion
- Infection: meningitis, brain abscess, encephalitis, septicaemia
- Endocrine: diabetic comas (hypoglycaemia, ketoacidosis, hyperosmolar non-ketotic coma, lactic acidosis), hypothyroidism, Addisonian crisis
- Metabolic: respiratory, hepatic and renal failure, severe hyponatraemia
- Neoplasm: primary or secondary brain tumours, malignant leptomeningeal infiltration

Table 12.2   Toxic-metabolic coma vs. coma due to structural brain lesions

Features	Toxic-metabolic	Structural
Clues to systemic illness	Usually present	Usually absent
Conscious state	Wax and wane	Stable
Respiration	Deep, frequent	Ataxic
Papilloedema	Usually absent	In mass lesion or SAH
Pupil size	Symmetrical, small, reactive	May be fixed or dilated

Table 12.2   (continued)

Features	Toxic-metabolic	Structural
Eye movement	Symmetrical, roving	Asymmetrical
Doll's eye	Usually intact	May be absent
Myoclonus	Associated with hypoxia	Absent
Focal deficits	Usually absent or fluctuating	Yes

Differential diagnosis

Persistent vegetative state is associated with extensive cortical grey and subcortical white matter lesions, but with preservation of sufficient brainstem function to sustain a vegetative state. It follows recovery from a comatose state and persists for more than a month. The most common causes are extensive traumatic head injury (e.g., road traffic accident, gunshot wound) and anoxic-ischaemic brain damage (e.g., cardiorespiratory arrest). Other causes include strokes, severe intracranial infections, metabolic encephalopathies, and neurodegenerative disorders at the terminal stage.

Following recovery from coma, the eyes open in response to pain initially and then to less noxious stimuli. When the sleep-wake cycle is established, the eyes open in the 'wakeful' periods. The term 'wakeful coma' refers to wakefulness without awareness. They may even blink to a visual threat or bright light, but there is no sustained tracking or consistent attempt to respond to visual stimuli. Vegetative functions (e.g., chewing, yawning, sucking, gagging, coughing) and brainstem reflexes are present. The patients are usually mute and have no self-awareness. Loud noises may provoke more complex brainstem responses, e.g., eye opening and grimacing. However, the cognitive functions are lost with no behavioural response to external stimuli.

These patients require long-term supportive care, including respiratory and nutritional support. Nursing care should be undertaken to prevent pressure sores, aspiration pneumonia, contractures, exposure keratitis, parotitis, urinary tract infection, and constipation. The family has to be given time to adjust to the situation and be encouraged to participate in the management.

Because of the long-term complications, life expectancy of these patients is substantially reduced, although some may survive for a longer time. This unfortunate state imposes a great burden on the family in many ways, e.g., psychological and financial. It also raises difficult ethical and medicolegal problems, for example whether to withdraw support or to intervene when the patient develops a severe infection or other complications. There is no easy answer. The cause of the vegetative state, the views and wishes of the family, and in some cases an advance directive, have to be taken into consideration.

Minimally conscious state refers to the condition in which the patient shows minimal but definite evidence of awareness despite profound cognitive impairment. Such evidence includes one or more of the following behaviours:
–   Simple command following
–   Gestural or verbal 'yes/no' responses (regardless of accuracy)
–   Intelligible verbalization
–   Purposeful behaviour including movements or affective behaviours in contingent relation to relevant stimuli; examples include:

Patients emerging from the vegetative state often enter into the minimally conscious state, which may be the end-point of their improvement, or a staging post on the way to further recovery.

Locked-in syndrome is due to a bilateral ventral pontine lesion. The patient is tetraplegic with lower cranial nerve palsies, but is alert and aware of the environment, and able to understand and communicate with eye closure and eye movements. A common cause is basilar artery occlusion.

Akinetic mutism is due to lesions in the frontal lobe bilaterally, midbrain or periventricular grey matter. Its causes include stroke, encephalitis, demyelinating disorders, and anoxic-ischaemic brain damage. The patient appears to be awake and the eyes may track moving objects, but there is no cognitive function or awareness. The sleep-wake cycles and respiratory functions are preserved.

Catatonia is characterized by mutism with markedly reduced motor activity, prolonged maintenance of posture with preserved ability to stand or sit. It is usually associated with a psychiatric disorder, e.g., schizophrenia, but may be due to a frontal lobe dysfunction or drug effect. The patient is both awake and aware with behavioural responsiveness markedly diminished.

Narcolepsy is a chronic disorder of excessive sleepiness with onset usually during adolescence or early adulthood. The clinical tetrad consists of:

- Daytime sleepiness: transient sleep attacks with interruption of normal daily activities (e.g., conversation, driving) which is potentially dangerous; having brief naps may help.
- Cataplexy: brief attacks of hypotonia or weakness, precipitated by laughter or anger
- Sleep paralysis: brief paralysis during transition from sleep to waking or vice versa
- Hypnagogic hallucinations: frightening visual, auditory or movement perceptions at sleep onset

The diagnosis is established by a positive multiple sleep latency test together with a normal sleep study. The latter excludes other conditions which may produce excessive daytime sleepiness, e.g., obstructive sleep apnoea. The latencies of both sleep onset (less than 10 minutes) and rapid eye movement (REM) onset (less than 20 minutes) are characteristically reduced. The presence of HLA-DR2 coded on chromosome 6 is strongly associated with narcolepsy. Central stimulants (e.g., methylphenidate, modafinil), together with daytime naps are effective strategies in maintaining daytime alertness. Tricyclics or selective serotonin reuptake inhibitors may be used to treat REM-related symptoms, hallucinations or sleep paralysis.

Diagnosis and management of comatose patients

Coma is a medical emergency. Delay in diagnosis and treatment increases mortality and morbidity.

1. Look for clinical clues of underlying causes (non-CNS, focal or diffuse CNS).
2. Investigations depend on the provisional clinical diagnosis.

3. Emergency measures (especially when there are few clues):
   - Maintain airway and institute ventilatory support if indicated.
   - Check haemoglucostix and give IV 50% glucose.
   - IV thiamine, IV naloxone, IV flumazenil
   - Blood and urine for toxicology screen, ABG, blood counts, and biochemistry
   - Consult the neurologist if indicated
4. General and supportive treatments
   - Frequent monitoring of neurological status and vital signs
   - Care of tracheostomy
   - Adequate nutrition and hydration
   - Treat systemic infection, e.g., pneumonia, urinary tract infection.
   - Care of incontinence
   - Prevention and care of bedsores
5. Specific treatment according to the cause of coma

Coma after cardiac arrest

Cerebral blood flow during resuscitation attains only 2–10% of pre-arrest values. Different organs tolerate ischaemia differently. For the brain, damage ensues when ischaemia exceeds five minutes. Coma is common following anoxic-ischaemic insult.

Neurological syndromes after cardiac arrest

Transient CNS deficit (< 12 hours) consists of confusion followed by antegrade amnesia. The prognosis is good, often with rapid complete recovery.

Persistent focal CNS deficit (> 12 hours)
- The cerebral syndrome is characterized by focal or multiple cortical infarcts especially at boundary zones. Amnesia, dementia, tetraparesis, cortical blindness, seizures, ataxia, myoclonus, and parkinsonism are common features. Recovery is slow and often incomplete.
- The spinal cord syndrome is characterized by focal or multifocal infarcts especially at boundary zones. The sequelae include

flaccid tetraparesis or paraparesis, urinary retention, and dissociated sensory loss (preserved touch and position). Recovery is
incomplete or minimal.

Global CNS damage usually results in persistent vegetative state
or brain death.

Management of coma after cardiac arrest

Maintain euglycaemia to avoid cerebral lactic acidosis. Avoid
factors which increase ICP. Monitoring of ICP may be necessary.
Raised ICP may be treated with:
- Sedatives ± neuromuscular blockers
- Mechanical hyperventilation
- Osmotic diuresis
- Steroids and barbiturates are not recommended

Achieve stable haemodynamics to ensure cerebral perfusion.
Commence standard treatment for seizures and watch out for status
epilepticus. Post-anoxic myoclonus may mimic status epilepticus.

Brain death

Guidelines for diagnosis

The prerequisites are:
1. The patient is in deep coma and requires mechanical ventilation
   because of cessation of spontaneous respiration. Cerebral and
   brainstem functions are absent.
2. There is irreversible brain damage. Cessation of all brain functions persists for an appropriate period (usually 24 hours) and
   the cause (e.g., massive cerebral haemorrhage or severe head
   injury) is established.
3. Complicating conditions which may mimic brain death have
   been excluded:
   - Drug intoxication and metabolic disturbance: Death should
     not be declared until the intoxicant has been removed, and
     metabolic abnormalities corrected, if possible.

- Hypothermia: Neurological testing is invalid if there is significant hypothermia, e.g., below 32°C. The body temperature must be above 35°C.
- Children: The recovery potential is higher compared to adults. A longer period of observation is desirable, especially in children below age 5 years.
- Shock: Clinical examination is unreliable in shock because of cerebral hypoperfusion. The systolic pressure should be at least 90 mmHg before testing for brain death.

Having satisfied these prerequisites, proceed to look for evidence of absent brainstem reflexes (Table 12.3). Care must be taken to exclude conditions which may interfere with interpretation of brainstem reflexes (Table 12.4). The steps in declaring brain death are presented schematically in Figure 12.1.

Table 12.3   Absence of brainstem reflexes in brain death

Brainstem reflexes	In brain death
Pupillary	Pupils fixed but not necessarily widely dilated
Corneal	No eye blink on touching the cornea
Oculocephalic	No eye movement on head turning
Oculovestibular	No eye movement to warm/cold saline irrigation to ears
Oropharyngeal	No gag/cough reflex during endotracheal suction
Respiratory	No ventilatory effort to apnoeic oxygenation with $PaCO_2 > 6.6$ kPa

Table 12.4   Conditions which may interfere with testing of brainstem reflexes

Pupillary reflexes	Local eye disease, e.g., cataract Atropine given during cardiac arrest
Oculovestibular reflexes	Local disease of ear canals AEDs, antidepressants, ototoxic antibiotics, alcohol, neuromuscular blockers
Respiratory reflexes	Post-hyperventilation apnoea Neuromuscular blockers, AEDs antidepressants
All brainstem reflexes	Barbiturates, other CNS depressants

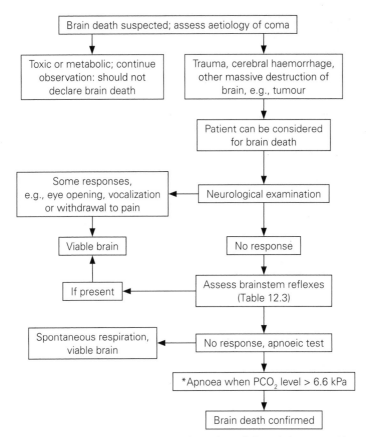

Figure 12.1   Flow chart for diagnosis of brain death

*These observations are usually repeated after an interval of 4 to 24 hours to avoid observer error.

Absent cortical activity (no EEG activity or cerebral blood flow) is not mandatory in the diagnosis of brainstem death. It should, however, be noted that EEG may be preserved in pure brainstem death, e.g., following basilar artery occlusion. Angiography, SPECT, transcranial Doppler, and perfusion CT brain may provide supporting evidence but are not mandatory.

Spinal cord reflexes may persist after brain death. Seizures and decerebrate or decorticate posturing are inconsistent with brain death.

The transplant team must not be involved in declaring brain death in potential organ donors. Brain death is to be certified by clinicians with experience in ICU or acute medical wards, and neurologists should be consulted if in doubt.

Living will

Since patients who are terminally ill, irreversibly comatose or mentally incapacitated can have their lives prolonged substantially through life-sustaining care, provision is available for individuals to issue an advance directive. This is a written document that gives the individuals the right to provide explicit instructions as to treatment preferences or rejection of treatment before they lose the decision-making capacity.

13 Infections of the Central Nervous System

Most CNS infections are neurological emergencies and require urgent medical attention. There are several features which distinguish CNS from systemic infections.

- The CNS is protected by the blood-brain-barrier.
- Penetration of the blood-brain-barrier is poor for many antimicrobial agents.
- Within the cranium, space for expansion is limited. Mass lesions and accompanying cerebral oedema may cause damage and herniation of brain parenchyma, resulting in significant morbidity and mortality.
- Neurological damage is mediated by various mechanisms often acting in concert (Figure 13.1).

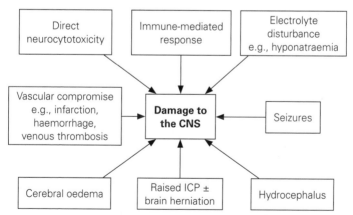

Figure 13.1   Mechanisms of neurological damage due to CNS infections

TYPES OF INFECTION

Meningitis

Meningitis refers to inflammation of the leptomeninges. The major cause is infection. Other causes of meningitis include the presence of blood in the subarachnoid space, neoplastic infiltration, and drugs (e.g., intrathecal contrast medium). Meningism refers to clinical features similar to meningitis but without evidence of inflammation.

Table 13.1   Likely pathogens in various susceptible populations and conditions

Susceptible population/condition	Pathogens
Neonates	coliforms (especially *E. coil*), group B streptococcus, *Listeria monocytogenes*
Infants	*H. influenzae*, meningococcus (*N. meningitidis*), pneumococcus (*Strep. pneumoniae*)
Young children and adults	meningococcus, pneumococcus
Older adults	pneumococcus
Elderly	pneumococcus, coliforms, *L. monocytogenes*
Immune deficiency	any organism: pneumococcus, coliforms, *L. monocytogenes*, staphylococci fungi (*Cryptococcal neoformans*, candida species, aspergillus, mucormycetes), parasitic (toxoplasma)
Indwelling CSF shunt	*Staph. aureus, Staph. epidermidis*
Neurosurgery	coliforms
Penetrating skull trauma, CSF rhinorrhoea postsplenectomy, sickle-cell disease	pneumococcus

Clinical features

The onset may be acute or insidious. Non-specific symptoms (headache, fever, chills, malaise, and lethargy) may be present in the early stage, followed by worsening headache, photophobia, nausea, and vomiting. Meningeal irritation results in spasms of neck extensors (neck rigidity) and hamstring muscles (Kernig's sign). Agitation and confusion may ensue. A high index of suspicion is required, especially at the extremes of age and in the immunocompromised, because these classical features may be inconspicuous.

Pyogenic meningitis

Cases with complications (e.g., seizures, septic shock, stupor, coma, and DIC) have a high morbidity and mortality. Features of raised ICP may develop. Focal signs (e.g., hemiparesis) may be due to infarction, abscess formation or subdural collection. Neurological sequelae (e.g., impaired higher mental functions, spasticity, cranial nerve palsies, deafness, ataxia, seizures, and hydrocephalus) are common. In recurrent bacterial meningitis, there is often CSF communication to the exterior, e.g., through neurosurgical procedures, CSF shunts, cribriform plate fracture. Pneumococcus and *H. influenzae* are the usual pathogens.

Chronic meningitis

This is commonly due to tuberculous or cryptococcal infection (*vide infra*).

Viral meningitis

It usually presents with meningism and is mostly benign. It also produces non-specific 'flu-like' symptoms, diarrhoea, myalgia, parotitis, and exanthemata. If focal signs appear, focal brain lesions (e.g., encephalitis and cerebral abscess) have to be excluded. The outcome is excellent with complete recovery in 1–2 weeks in most cases. Enteroviruses (e.g., coxsackievirus A and B, echoviruses) account for more than 75% of cases. It spreads via the faecal-oral route and is common in young children. Other viruses include paramyxoviruses (mumps, measles), herpes viruses (Epstein-Barr, herpes simplex virus), and arenavirus (lymphocytic choriomeningitis).

Complications (mainly of pyogenic and chronic meningitis)

- Basal meningeal adhesions (e.g., in TBM) are due to incomplete organization of inflammatory exudates. It is associated with raised ICP, hydrocephalus (due to meningeal adhesions or dural sinus thrombosis) and cranial nerve palsies. The III, IV, and VI cranial nerves are most often affected. VIII nerve damage tends to persist.
- Cerebral infarction due to arterial and venous sinus thrombosis.
- Poor concentration, intellectual impairment, and mental retardation. Cerebral palsy can complicate infantile and childhood meningitis.
- Seizures complicate 10% of patients with acute bacterial meningitis. About 5% develop epilepsy.
- Extension of infection may cause cerebritis, cerebral abscess, subdural effusion or empyema.
- SIADH and other electrolyte disturbances.

Investigations

- CBC, ESR, clotting profile, CXR
- Culture (blood, sputum, urine, throat and nasal swabs)
- Skull X-ray (if sinusitis, mastoditis or CSF rhinorrhoea suspected)
- CT/MRI brain in all cases
- CSF analysis is essential in all cases of suspected neurological infections unless contraindications are present (see Chapter 2).

CSF analysis should include routine microscopy, protein, glucose (with simultaneous blood glucose), Gram stain, culture and sensitivity, AFB smear and cultures, Indian ink stain for cryptococcal capsule, and antigen detection for cryptococcus. Antigen detection for *H. influenzae*, meningococcus, pneumococcus and listeria, and PCR for mycobacterium are indicated when specific microorganisms are suspected. The CSF opening pressure should be checked. Repeat CSF examination may be required for monitoring therapeutic response. The abnormal CSF patterns are listed in Table 13.2.

Table 13.2   CSF findings in different infections

Type of infection	CSF findings
Pyogenic meningitis	Marked increase in WBC (neutrophils) and protein, decrease in glucose
Partially treated bacterial meningitis	Increase in WBC (neutrophil predominant) and protein, decreased or normal glucose
Viral meningitis/encephalitis	Increase in WBC (lymphocyte) and protein, normal glucose
Chronic meningitis (TB and fungal)	Increase in WBC (lymphocyte) and protein, decrease in glucose
Extrameningeal infections (cerebral, epidural or subdural abscess)	Increase in WBC (neutrophil predominant) and protein, normal glucose

Encephalitis

Encephalitis and myelitis refer to inflammation of parenchyma of the brain and spinal cord respectively, and may coexist with meningitis (meningoencephalomyelitis). Most cases are due to viruses which can damage the CNS in two ways: direct invasion of host cells, or post-infectious immune-mediated damage to the brain/spinal cord (see Chapter 9). There is great variability in the clinical presentation. In many cases, the virus cannot be identified.

Causes

Acute viral encephalitis

Epidemic viral encephalitis is mostly due to arboviruses (e.g., alphavirus, flavivirus, and bunyavirus) which are tick- or mosquito-borne. Japanese B encephalitis is the most common cause worldwide. Other causes include dengue fever and influenza.

Sporadic viral encephalitis occurs as a primary infection or follows reactivation. The common causes include herpes viruses (HSV-1 and -2, varicella-zoster, Epstein-Barr virus, CMV), para-myxoviruses (measles, mumps, rubella), retroviruses (HIV), and enteroviruses (coxsackie viruses, echoviruses, polioviruses).

The pathological lesions tend to be diffuse, but HSV affects particularly the temporal and frontal lobes. Characteristic changes include perivascular infiltration of lymphocytes and plasma cells, neuronophagia (dead or infected neurones engulfed by microglia), and viral inclusion bodies (e.g., in rabies, HSV encephalitis).

Non-viral encephalitis

Rickettsia (typhus, scrub typhus, Rocky Mountain spotted fever), *Plasmodium falciparum* (cerebral malaria), *Toxoplasma gondii*, Trypanosomiasis (American and African sleeping sickness), *Acanthamoeba* (amoebiasis), *L. monocytogenes* (listeriosis), *Borrelia burgdorferi* (Lyme disease) may also cause encephalitis.

Post-infectious encephalitis (see Chapter 9)

Clinical features

Prodromal symptoms of systemic infection, e.g., fever, headache, nausea, and general malaise, are often present. Altered mental state and seizures (often serial or status) are common presenting features. Other clinical manifestations include memory deficit, dysphasia, agnosia, visual disturbance, limb weakness, and myoclonus. In children with varicella-zoster encephalitis, cerebellar ataxia is a characteristic feature.

Differential diagnosis

- Bacterial meningitis complicated by cerebral abscess, oedema or venous thrombosis

- Metabolic encephalopathy, e.g., drug overdose, hypoglycaemia, renal or liver failure, hyponatraemia
- Complex partial status epilepticus from other causes

Investigations

- MRI/CT brain or spinal cord may show oedema and localized
areas of necrosis.
- CSF analysis including virus cultures and HSV-PCR
- Paired serum viral titres; urine, stools, throat swab samples for
viral studies
- EEG shows diffuse slow wave and spike activity. A temporal
focus may be seen in HSV encephalitis.
- Brain biopsy is seldom necessary.

Slow virus CNS infections

These syndromes include Creutzfeldt-Jakob disease (see Chapter 11),
progressive multifocal leukoencephalopathy (PML) and subacute
sclerosing panencephalitis (SSPE).

PML is a subacute demyelinating opportunistic infection
caused by the JC virus, a DNA-containing papovavirus. Most
cases are related to HIV-1 infected patients (about 2% of AIDS
patients develop PML). Patients on long-term immunosuppression
(e.g., liver or renal transplants, SLE, lymphoproliferative disease)
are also at risk. It is associated with progressive multifocal neurological signs, seizures, personality change, and dementia. There is
no effective treatment. Prognosis is poor with death within weeks
or months. Rarely there may be spontaneous remission.

SSPE is a rare progressive chronic demyelinating illness associated with preceding measles infection. It mainly affects children. The onset is insidious with gradual deterioration of school
performance. It progresses with development of neurological
signs (cerebellar ataxia, myoclonic jerks, seizures), eventually to
a mute, stuporous, and rigid state with autonomic instability. CSF
and serum may show raised measles antibody titres. EEG shows
repetitive, high amplitude, slow wave discharges alternating with

periods of little or no activity (burst-suppression pattern). There is no specific treatment. Prognosis is poor and death occurs within 1–3 years.

Abscess involving the brain and spinal cord

Intracerebral abscess

For an abscess to develop in previously normal brain tissue, some degree of focal cerebral ischaemia is probably necessary; hence the less vascularized sites (e.g., the white matter, junction of white and grey matter) tend to be affected. Inflammation begins with localized cerebritis followed by liquefaction, necrosis, and abscess formation. Brain abscesses are then encapsulated and surrounded by further cerebritis and oedema.

Subdural abscess/empyema

It is a fulminating purulent infection located between the dura and the pia-arachnoid membranes. The source of infection is usually identifiable (e.g., from paranasal sinuses). Thrombophlebitis of the cortical veins is a frequent complication which can result in cortical infarction (see Chapter 6). Major dural sinus thrombosis may also occur.

Spinal abscess

It can be intramedullary or epidural. Most cases are due to haematogenous spread. They present with back pain and features of acute cord lesion.

Routes of infection and predisposing factors

- Direct spread from adjacent infection (e.g., sinusitis, otitis media, mastoiditis). Chronic otitis media is probably the most common source of infection.

- Direct external penetration of CSF space (e.g., craniofacial trauma, penetrating wound of skull, indwelling CSF shunts)
- Haematogenous spread from dental infection, lung abscess, bronchiectasis, pneumonia, osteomyelitis, cardiovascular disorders (e.g., endocarditis, right-to-left shunt), IV drug abuse
- Immune deficiency (e.g., HIV, hyposplenism, sickle cell disease, drug-induced)
- Complications arising from acute bacterial meningitis
- Post-cerebral irradiation, e.g., NPC

Clinical features

- Systemic features: fever, chills, rigours, decreased peripheral perfusion
- Raised ICP: headache, vomiting, depressed consciousness, papilloedema
- Focal signs and symptoms are present in 75% of cases. The most common site is the temporal lobe followed by the frontal lobe. They may be multiple and occasionally isolated in the cerebellum. Focal deficits include hemiplegia, dysphasia, and visual field defects.
- Meningitis is a rare complication and is associated with a poor prognosis. It develops after rupture of the abscess into ventricles and subarachnoid space.
- Seizures occur in up to 30% of cases, more often for abscesses in the frontal lobe than the temporal lobe.

Microbiology

In most cases, two or more microorganisms can be identified, depending on the anatomical site and underlying cause. In HIV cases, *Toxoplasma gondii* is the most common pathogen.
- Bacterial:
  Usually polymicrobial (mixed aerobic and anaerobic)

  Aerobes: *Strep. milleri* or *pneumoniae*, *Staph. aureus*, Gram negative bacilli (pseudomonas, coliforms)

  Anaerobes: *Bacteriodes fragilis*, fusobacterium, pepto-streptococcus, peptococcus, actinomyces, nocardia

- Other pathogens:
  Fungi: cryptococcus, aspergillus
  Protozoa: *Toxoplasma gondii* (HIV-related), *Entamoeba histolytica*
  Parasites: *Taenia solium* (cysticercosis), echinococcus (hydatid cyst), *Strongyloides stercoralis* (strongyloidiasis)

Complications

- Gliosis (scarring) of brain resulting in an increased risk of epilepsy
- Herniation of brain especially in posterior fossa abscess
- Rupture of abscess into the subarachnoid space and ventricles
- Residual focal neurological deficits
- Recurrence of brain abscess

Investigations

- Neuroimaging is the mainstay of investigations. Although CSF is usually abnormal, LP is contraindicated because of the risk of coning.
- CT brain (plain and contrast): brain abscess typically shows ring enhancement with contrast.
- MRI brain is the investigation of choice. It is more sensitive in differentiating the various pathological components of the abscess. T_1 weighted images show the hypointense central purulent material and contrast-enhanced hyperintense capsule; T_2 weighted images show the hyperintense surrounding oedema.
- Microbiological investigations: blood cultures and cultures from suspected sources of sepsis, e.g., pus from abscess
- Search for underlying foci: CXR, echocardiogram, ENT examination, X-ray of the sinuses
- EEG is of little value in diagnosis but may be useful in documenting seizure activity.

Prognosis

The overall mortality has declined markedly with the advent of modern neuroimaging and antibiotics. Prognosis is poor when the abscess has ruptured, is in the posterior fossa, or is not responsive to aspiration and antibiotic therapy.

Treatment of CNS infections

General principles

1. The infective focus should be sought as it is a guide to empirical therapy.
2. Sepsis screen especially blood culture should be done immediately, preferably prior to starting antibiotic therapy. However, if meningococcal septicaemia is suspected, IV penicillin should be started immediately.
3. LP should not be delayed unless there are features of raised ICP or focal neurological deficits, bleeding tendency or suspected brain abscess.
4. Empirical therapy should be started without waiting for the culture or CSF results. IV antimicrobial agents should be given in adequate doses.
5. Supportive therapy involves maintenance of airway and tissue perfusion, correction of dehydration, electrolyte disturbance and hypoxaemia, as well as AED therapy.
6. All patients should be monitored regularly for complications (e.g., cerebral oedema, septic shock, DIC), and they should be nursed in a high dependency or ICU setting.
7. There should be close liaison with microbiologists to facilitate immediate reporting of results and management of poor responders.
8. Steroids may be given to reduce inflammatory tissue damage.

Antimicrobial therapy

Pyogenic meningitis

The empirical regime is IV benzylpenicillin and a third-generation cephalosporin, e.g., ceftriaxone, ceftazidime, cefotaxime. In suspected shunt infection or meningitis following cranial trauma or neurosurgery, IV vancomycin is added to cover methicillin-resistant *Staph. epidermidis*. The antibiotic regime should then be modified according to the culture and sensitivity results (Table 13.3).

Table 13.3 Antibiotic regime based on the infecting organism

Organism	Antimicrobial therapy
N. meningitidis *H. influenzae*	(1) Benzylpenicillin (2) Third-generation cephalosporin
Strep. pneumoniae	(1) Benzylpenicillin ± third-generation cephalosporin (2) Vancomycin if methicillin-resistant
Strep. suis	Benzylpenicillin
Group B streptococcus	(1) Cloxacillin ± rifampicin (2) Cefuroxime (3) Vancomycin ± rifampicin, if methicillin-resistant (4) Septrin (± rifampicin) for some strains
Gram negative bacilli (*E. Coli*, klebsiella, pseudomonas, enterobacter acinetobacter, citrobacter, serratia, salmonella, proteus)	Broad spectrum penicillin (ticarcillin, mezlocillin, piperacillin) ± third-generation cephalosporin ± aminoglycoside
Anaerobes (*Bacteroides fragilis*, peptostreptococcus, fusobacterium)	Metronidazole
L. monocytogenes	Benzylpenicillin + aminoglycoside

Viral encephalitis

IV acyclovir is effective against herpes viruses. It should be started as soon as possible if encephalitis is clinically suspected. If CMV infection is specifically suspected, IV ganciclovir should be used.

Intracerebral abscess

- Eradicate the abscess and the source of infection. Antibiotic treatment (IV benzylpenicillin and cefotaxime) is often started empirically. IV metronidazole is added if the abscess is associated with ENT infection, or located in the frontal or temporal region. The regime is modified according to the culture results and continued for at least 6 weeks. In abscesses from neurosurgical procedures or head injury, IV cloxacillin or vancomycin is added to cover *Staph. aureus*. Neurosurgery is required in some cases. The procedures include aspiration and excision of the abscess.
- Mannitol infusion is used to lower raised ICP.
- Prophylactic AED may be given at the time of diagnosis because up to 30% of patients develop seizures.

CNS infections in immunocompromised hosts

General principles

There is a growing population of immunocompromised subjects as a result of disease (e.g., collagen vascular disease, lymphoproliferative disorders, malignancy, HIV infection), immunosuppressive therapy (steroids, cytotoxic drugs, irradiation), or more often a combination of disease activity and adverse events from therapy.

Haematogenous spread is the usual route and the primary source is often lung infection. Immunodeficiency state may allow reactivation of latent infection in the host.

Unusual infections or atypical presentation of common infections are often encountered. The general approach is similar to that for immunocompetent hosts but a high index of suspicion is required as classical signs of infection may be absent. Fever, headache, meningism, and altered consciousness should raise the possibility of CNS infection. Appropriate microbiological tests should be performed and empirical therapy in adequate dosage started as soon as possible. The choice of antimicrobial agents depends on the type of immunodeficiency, clinical presentation, and local prevalence of opportunistic infections.

Types of immunodeficiency

Asplenism/hyposplenism

The causes include post-splenectomy, sickle cell anaemia, and coeliac disease. These patients are prone to encapsulated bacterial infections, e.g., pneumococcal meningitis. Post-splenectomy patients require prophylactic penicillin and polyvalent pneumococcal vaccine.

Antibody deficiency

Patients with hypogammaglobulinaemia or lymphoproliferative diseases have antibody deficiency. They are prone to bacterial and viral infections.

Complement system deficiency

Complements are important amplifying factors for antibody-directed lysis of pathogens in the blood stream. Deficiency may be congenital (usually of specific components of the complement system), or acquired (e.g., systemic vasculitis). These patients are prone to develop meningococcaemia.

Neutropenia

The causes include chemotherapy, irradiation, and aplastic anaemia. These patients are prone to opportunistic bacterial and fungal infections. The risk increases significantly when the neutrophil count is less than 0.5×10^9/l.

Cell-mediated immune deficiency

Cell-mediated immunity is directed mainly against intracellular pathogens. The cause may be congenital (e.g., Di George syndrome, severe combined immunodeficiency) or acquired (e.g., HIV infection, lymphoproliferative disorders, malignancies, immunosuppressive therapy). These patients are prone to viral, parasitic, mycobacterial, and listerial infections, as well as reactivation of latent infections.

Patients with AIDS, renal, and bone marrow transplant are increasingly encountered. They are prone to a variety of CNS infections which are summarized in Table 13.4.

SELECTED ENTITIES

Meningococcal (*Neisseria meningitidis*) meningitis

It is the most common form of meningitis worldwide, affecting mainly young adults and children. It has a short incubation period, often preceded by upper respiratory tract infection or diarrhoeal illness. The onset is fulminating, and meningeal signs may be absent. Petechial haemorrhages or purpuric skin lesions occur in about half of the cases. It may progress rapidly to coma, septic shock, DIC, and adrenal haemorrhage (Waterhouse-Friederichsen syndrome). Carriers are usually asymptomatic and infection is spread by droplets. IV benzylpenicillin is the treatment of choice.

Streptococcal suis meningitis

It is a common cause of bacterial meningitis in adults in Hong Kong. It is associated with exposure to pigs or pork products. Infection is usually through skin wounds followed by haematogenous spread. Early and permanent deafness due to cochlear damage is common. IV benzylpenicillin is the treatment of choice.

Table 13.4 CNS infections in three groups of immunocompromised patients

Pathogens	AIDS	Renal transplant	Bone marrow transplant

Viral	CMV encephalitis
	PML
	AIDS-dementia complex
	HIV meningitis
		CMV encephalitis
		PML
		HSV and varicella-zoster
		  meningoencephalitis
		EBV encephalitis
			HSV and varicella-zoster
			  meningoencephalitis
			CMV encephalitis (rare)

Bacterial	TBM nocardia intracerebral abscess	listerial meningitis TBM or TB abscess atypical mycobacterial infection	listerial meningitis
Fungal	cryptococcosis candidiasis aspergillosis	cryptococcosis candidiasis mucormycosis aspergillosis	aspergillosis (brain abscess or diffuse meningoencephalitis)
Protozoal	toxoplasmosis (most common)	toxoplasmosis *Pneumocystis carinii*	toxoplasmosis (rare)

Dengue fever

It is an arthropod-borne infection endemic in tropical and subtropical regions. The dengue virus belongs to the family of *Flaviviridae*, which are single-stranded RNA viruses. The mosquito vector is primarily *Aedes aegypti*, which breeds in polluted waters. Dengue infections can be asymptomatic or manifests with fever, haemorrhagic fever, and septic shock syndrome. The patient presents with intermittent high fever, severe retro-orbital headaches, myalgia, arthralgia, vomiting, and abdominal pain. Its complications include massive bleeding due to DIC and thrombocytopaenia, myocarditis, and liver failure. Encephalitis and metabolic encephalopathy may occur, and focal neurological deficits and meningism may be present. During the febrile stage, dengue viruses may be isolated from blood and other tissue samples. Dengue-specific IgM and IgG enzyme-linked immunosorbent assays (ELISA) aids the diagnosis. Treatment is symptomatic and supportive.

Zika virus infection

It is an arthropod-borne infection resembling dengue fever, and is endemic in tropical and subtropical regions. It is transmitted by the mosquito vector *Aedes* species. Non-symptomatic infections are very common. Symptoms, if present, include a maculopapular rash, fever, headaches, and joint pains. The major health concern is for pregnant women because of *in utero* transmission. A variety of neurological disorders including microcephaly in the baby and GBS in the patient are associated with this infection. Serological diagnosis is similar to dengue fever. In acutely ill patients, Zika virus can be identified by reverse transcription-polymerase chain reaction (RT-PCR) of their serum, saliva or urine.

Herpes simplex encephalitis

HSV-1 causes more than 95% of adult herpes encephalitis. It also causes cold sores and herpetic whitlows. It occurs as a primary infection or follows reactivation from the trigeminal ganglion or brain. It has a predilection for the temporal and frontal lobes.

HSV-2 encephalitis may be acquired by the neonate from the mother's genital tract during delivery.

Adults have a prodromal phase with headache, malaise, respiratory symptoms, and vomiting for a few days, followed by increasing drowsiness, confusion, hallucination, epileptic seizures, and coma. Focal cortical signs may be present, e.g., aphasia and hemiparesis.

EEG shows focal or epileptic activity in about 60% of cases, especially over the frontal and temporal regions. CSF shows lymphocytic pleocytosis with raised protein and normal glucose. HSV-PCR may be positive in blood and CSF samples. CT brain is usually normal but may show subtle changes (Figure 13.2a). MRI brain may show T_2-weighted hyperintense lesion (from oedema) in the temporal or frontal lobes (Figure 13.2b).

Acyclovir must be given IV in adequate dosage and duration (10 mg/kg q8h for 10 days). Steriods may be given concomitantly if there is significant cerebral oedema. Seizures should be promptly controlled with AED. HSV encephalitis has a high mortality (50–70%) if left untreated.

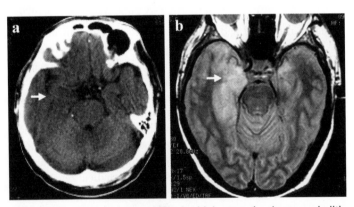

Figure 13.2   CT brain (a) in a patient with herpes simplex encephalitis with the arrow pointing at subtle swelling of the right temporal lobe. MRI brain (b) performed around the same time in the same patient showing bilateral temporal lobe swelling with hyper-intense signals in the mesial temporal regions on a proton-density image; changes were more marked in the right temporal lobe (arrow).

Varicella-zoster (VZV) infection

The VZV (Herpes virus) causes two syndromes:
- Varicella (chicken-pox) is usually a self-limiting primary infection with a vesicular rash.
- Zoster (shingles) is caused by reactivation of the latent virus resulting in dermatomal vesicular skin lesions.

The neurological complications of VZV are more likely to develop in immunocompromised patients. The relatively common complications are:
- Cerebellar ataxia is the most common neurological complication of chickenpox. It usually affects children. The ataxia usually occurs at the onset of skin rash, and is accompanied by fever, vomiting, headaches, and meningism. The ataxia usually resolves completely within 3 weeks.
- Post-herpetic neuralgia describes the chronic dermatomal neuralgia that persists after the herpetic skin eruption has healed. It is more likely to develop in the elderly, and varies in intensity from mild paraesthesia to severe sharp pain.
- Cranial neuropathies (e.g., Ramsay-Hunt syndrome, which is caused by reactivation of VZV in the external auditory canal with ensuing damage to the ipsilateral facial nerve and facial palsy)

Uncommon complications include:
- Encephalitis which presents with fever, altered consciousness, and seizures about a week after the onset of the skin rash. EEG may show epileptiform or slow-wave activity. MRI brain initially shows T_2 weighted hyperintense, multiple lesions in the subcortical white matter. With progression, they can coalesce, cavitate, and spread to involve the cortical regions. CSF examination may show a high opening pressure, lymphocytic pleocytosis, elevated protein with normal glucose, and VZV on PCR. Untreated VZV encephalitis is usually fatal. Antiviral treatment should be given early.
- Leukoencephalopathy
- Aseptic meningitis
- Transverse myelitis

- Peripheral neuropathies. Segmental motor neuropathies affecting cranial and peripheral motor nerves can result in weakness of the affected myotome.

Treatment of VZV infection consists of:
- skin care and prevention of secondary bacterial skin infections
- symptomatic relief for pain (e.g., pregabalin, gabapentin, amitriptyline, NSAID)
- oral antiviral drugs for VZV infections include acyclovir, valaciclovir (prodrug of acyclovir) and famciclovir (prodrug of penciclovir). IV acyclovir is required in severe infections especially in immunocompromised patients.

Prevention of herpes zoster infection and related post-herpetic neuralgia for individuals over age 50 years can be achieved with a single SC dose of zoster live vaccine.

Japanese B encephalitis

The causative agent is an arbovirus, and the mosquito vector is mainly *Culex tritaeniorhynchus*. The infection is amplified in birds and pigs, and is endemic in tropical and subtropical regions. Japanese B encephalitis presents with fever and headache associated with aseptic meningitis and encephalitis. The encephalitis is of rapid onset, manifesting with psychosis, seizures, extrapyramidal signs, and focal neurological deficits. Convalescence can be prolonged, and is characterized by persistent weakness, ataxia, and emotional lability. Serological tests are used for diagnosis. Treatment is supportive. Tourists travelling to endemic areas should consider vaccination.

Human immunodeficiency virus-1 (HIV-1) infection

The neurological manifestations in HIV are diverse. They include:
- meningitis
- HIV-induced encephalopathy (HIV-associated major cognitive/motor disorder; AIDS-Dementia Complex) typically occurs in the advanced immunodeficiency stage, but rarely may present

in the early stages. It is characterized by an insidious onset of cognitive dysfunction with loss of concentration, forgetfulness, and slow mentation. There may be other associated features, e.g., masked facies, hypophonia, bradykinesia, rigidity, and postural instability. MRI may show generalized cerebral atrophy with diffuse white matter T_2 weighted hyperintense lesions. It responds to anti-HIV treatment.

- Vascular myelopathy
- Peripheral neuropathy
- CNS opportunistic infections (see Table 13.4)
- Cancer (e.g., primary CNS lymphoma)
- Cerebral infarction
- Cerebral haemorrhage
- Drugs used in treating HIV-1 infection may cause peripheral neuropathy and myelopathy.

Tuberculosis of the CNS

It can occur in the form of TBM, tuberculoma, myelopathy, radic-ulopathy, and arachnoiditis. It is often associated with pulmonary or miliary TB.

TBM

It is caused by *Mycobacterium tuberculosis* in the majority of cases, and occasionally by *Mycobacterium bovis*.

Onset is insidious over several weeks. Symptoms are often non-specific and include vague headache, malaise, anorexia, inter-mittent low-grade fever, and night sweats. Meningism may be mild or absent. Choroid tubercles are common in children but rare in adults. Reduced consciousness, seizures, cranial nerve palsies, and coma may intervene.

The common CSF findings are listed in Table 13.2. It should be noted that neutrophil-predominant pleocytosis may be seen during the early phase of TBM. CT/MRI brain may show hyperintense meninges with contrast, hydrocephalus, cerebral infarction or tuberculoma (Figure 13.3).

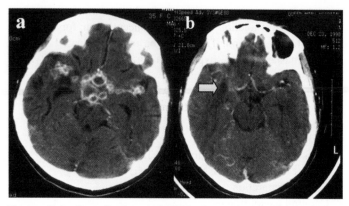

Figure 13.3 Complications of TBM. Contrast CT brain showing (a) marked basal meningeal enhancement and multiple tuberculomas, and (b) an acute cerebral infarct (arrow).

Treatment

1. Oral isoniazid 300–450 mg/day, rifampicin 600 mg/day, and pyrazinamide 1.5–2 g/day should be given for at least 9 months. Pyridoxine (50 mg/day) should be added to prevent isoniazid-induced neuropathy.
2. Ethambutol may also be given. Adherence to dosage recommendation and regular monitoring of visual acuity are required to pre-empt toxic optic neuropathy.
3. IM streptomycin may be given. Second-line drugs (e.g., capreomycin and cycloserine) are used if drug resistance develops or when first-line drugs produce unacceptable side effects.
4. Corticosteroid is indicated to reduce inflammation arising from TBM in those patients with complications such as elevated ICP, spinal block, impending intracerebral herniation, and extreme neurological compromise.

Tuberculoma

It can be found in any site within the brain parenchyma, but is commonly supratentorial in adults and infratentorial in children.

It may be solitary or multiple. It is a discrete mass with a caseating and necrotic core surrounded by granulation tissue. Tuberculoma can be calcified.

Clinical features

Signs of raised ICP and epileptic seizures are common. Fever, meningism, and malaise are uncommon.

Treatment

Drug therapy is the same as for TBM. Surgical decompression and excision may be required in cases of failed medical therapy or significantly raised ICP.

CNS fungal infections

They tend to cause severe neurological syndromes with chronic basal meningitis. Obstructive hydrocephalus is a frequent complication. Major pathogens are cryptococcus, coccidioides, candida, and histoplasma.

Cryptococcal meningitis

It is the most common form of fungal meningitis which is caused by *Cryptococcus neoformans*. This fungus is ubiquitous in the environment but is found in greater concentration in pigeon's droppings. Most cases develop in patients with cellular immune deficiency. Over half of the patients are immunocompromised.

Clinical features

The patient often presents with non-specific symptoms such as fever, headache, and irritability, followed by mental confusion, seizures, and cranial nerve palsies.

Diagnosis

CSF analysis typically shows high protein, lymphocyte-predominant pleocytosis, low glucose, positive Indian ink smear, and raised cryptococcal antigen titre. The serum cryptococcal antigen titre is also elevated.

Treatment

1. IV amphotericin B with concurrent flucytosine in the induction phase for an adequate period. Amphotericin B requires a test dose on the first administration as it can cause severe allergic reaction. It can also cause nephrotoxicity. The incorporation of amphotericin into liposomes alters the pharmacokinetics of the drug and significantly improves the tolerability profile compared to conventional amphotericin B.
2. After completion of the induction phase, a consolidation phase using oral fluconazole is usually given until the CSF findings have returned to normal.
3. Other regimes using a combination of IV amphotericin B and fluconazole have been used in the induction and consolidation phases.
4. Repeat CSF analyses are performed to monitor response to treatment.

Cerebral toxoplasmosis

It is caused by *Toxoplasma gondii* and is characterized by multi-focal cerebral abscesses with a predilection for the basal ganglia. Infection is generally due to reactivation of latent organism. The presentation is usually subacute with fever, impaired consciousness, seizures, and focal neurological deficits. A major differential diagnosis is primary cerebral lymphoma, which may also be found in cerebral AIDS. A stereotactic brain biopsy may be necessary especially if it is unresponsive to antimicrobial agents. Treatment consists of pyrimethamine and sulphadiazine for 4–6 weeks and is then maintained at lower doses. Folate supplement is given to prevent pyrimethamine-induced anaemia.

Spirochaetal diseases

These include leptospirosis, Lyme disease, neurosyphilis, and relapsing fever. Spirochaetes penetrate through skin or mucus membrane, disseminate in blood, and produce clinical disease in stages, separated by latent phases.

Lyme disease

It is endemic in North America and Europe. It is caused by *Borrelia burgdorferi*, which is borne by Ixodes ticks. Lyme disease is a multisystem and multistaged disease. Neurological involvement occurs in about 10–40% of symptomatic diseases. In the early stages, a mild 'flu-like' syndrome and erythema migrans develop. Later, septic meningitis, fluctuating headache, cranial neuritis (unilateral or bilateral facial palsy), asymmetrical painful radiculitis, and arthritis can intervene. If untreated, a persistent stage develops with chronic encephalopathy and axonal polyradiculoneuropathy.

The diagnosis depends on a high index of suspicion. Erythema migrans may develop at the site of tick bite in about 60–80% of cases. ELISA detection of *Borrelia burgdorferi* antibodies can be used, but false positives may occur in patients with leptospirosis or syphilis.

Treatment consists of IV ceftriaxone for 2–6 weeks. Alternatively, oral amoxycillin or doxycycline may be used for at least a month.

Neurosyphilis

Syphilis is a sexually transmitted disease caused by *Treponema pallidum*. CNS invasion may occur within a few weeks or months following the primary infection, but is usually asymptomatic at this stage. If left untreated, meningitis may develop, and about 10% develop tertiary (meningovascular syphilis) or late syphilis (general paralysis of the insane, tabes dorsalis, taboparesis).

Meningovascular syphilis

The clinical onset may be abrupt or gradual and occurs within 10 years of the primary infection. It may present with meningitis, CVD, isolated cranial nerve palsies (especially II, VI, VII, VIII), papilloedema, spinal cord syndromes, and hydrocephalus.

General paralysis of the insane (GPI)

GPI is a subacute progressive meningoencephalitis which occurs between 10 and 20 years after the primary infection. It presents with disturbance of higher mental functions, e.g., personality changes, delusion of grandeur, poor concentration, memory deficits, and loss of insight. Eventually, the patient becomes increasingly tetraparetic, incontinent, and dysarthric. Tabes dorsalis may coexist with GPI as taboparesis.

Tabes dorsalis

It usually presents between 10 and 25 years after the primary infection. Clinical features consist of lightning pain to the limbs, sensory ataxia, and bladder hypotonia. Associated features include Argyll Robertson pupils, visceral crisis, and Charcot's joint in the legs or lumbar spine. In the late stage, serum and CSF VDRL may be negative, but CSF TPHA remains positive and specific for neurosyphilis.

Treatment

Treatment in the early stages can often reverse the disease process. If treatment is delayed, progressive changes are only partially reversible. In active neurosyphilis, IM procaine penicillin is given with oral probenecid for 14 days. Prednisolone is given before penicillin to provide cover for the Herxheimer reaction (malaise, fever, headache, arthralgia). Oral erythromycin or deoxycycline can be given if the patient is allergic to penicillin. Repeated CSF analysis is required to monitor response after completion of therapy at

6 weeks' and 3 months' intervals. Lymphocytic pleocytosis should normalize within 3 months of initiation of treatment, and protein within 6 months. For symptomatic relief, lightning pain may be treated with carbamazepine and visceral crisis with subcutaneous adrenaline. Sexual contacts should be screened for syphilis.

Tetanus

It is a life-threatening condition caused by tetanospasmin (tetanus neurotoxin). The clinical picture is dominated by muscle spasms and autonomic dysfunction. The infection is acquired through a contaminated wound, especially deep puncture wounds or those which contain foreign materials. Spores of *Clostridium tetani* enter the wound site and germinate in anaerobic conditions. The toxin produced diffuses away from the wound to adjacent muscles (causing local tetanus) and the blood stream (causing generalized tetanus). It is taken up by peripheral nerve terminals. Once inside the nerve, the toxin moves to the anterior horn cells and into pre-synaptic nerve terminals of inhibitory interneurones in the spinal cord. The toxin then causes disinhibition of the motor neurones and sympathetic neurones.

Clinical features

The clinical features depend on the distribution of toxin. In generalized tetanus, muscle spasms are often seen in muscles innervated by short axons (pharyngeal and posterior spinal) and appear several hours later, followed by those with longer axons (limb and abdominal). Increased muscle tone and reflexes are the earliest signs, especially in the masseters (causing trismus), pharyngeal muscles (causing dysphagia, aspiration pneumonia), and posterior spinal muscles (causing stiff neck, opisthotonus). Later, contraction of facial muscles may draw back the angle of the mouth with pursing of the lips (risus sardonicus). Life-threatening laryngeal spasms and respiratory muscles involvement may intervene. Sympathetic symptoms (hypertension, tachycardia, simultaneous arteriolar and venous constriction, raised cardiac output) appear 3 or 4 days after the first muscular symptoms. This delay is due to the complex route which the toxin takes to reach the lateral horns of the spinal cord.

Specific treatment

- Antibiotics: IV benzylpenicillin and metronidazole for at least 5 days
- Tetanus antitoxin: IM human tetanus immunoglobulin to be given before debridement of any wound
- Active immunization with adsorbed tetanus toxoid (ATT) given to a limb where antitoxin was not given
- Wound management e.g., debridement of necrotic tissue

Symptomatic treatment

- Diazepam to reduce muscle tone and anxiety
- Neuromuscular blockers, e.g., alcuronium, pancuronium
- Tracheostomy, mechanical ventilation
- Correction of fluid and electrolyte imbalance, and maintenance of nutrition through nasogastric tube
- Treatment of sympathetic overactivity with labetalol or magnesium sulphate infusion

14 Spinal Cord Disorders

Spinal cord disorders or myelopathies frequently cause severe and permanent disability because the spinal cord contains the entire motor and sensory systems of the trunk and limbs. Therefore, prompt diagnosis and treatment are essential. In particular, acute spinal cord compression is a neurological emergency.

Classification

Spinal cord disorders may be classified according to their causes. Trauma is the most common cause of myelopathy. For acute non-traumatic myelopathies, transverse myelitis and cord compression are common whereas spinal cord stroke is rare. In chronic non-traumatic myelopathies, spondylosis and benign tumours account for most cases. Syringomyelia, multiple sclerosis, degenerative and paraneoplastic cord lesions should be considered in the differential diagnosis. Subacute combined degeneration of spinal cord and syphilitic myelitis are rare but treatable entities.

Congenital and developmental disorders

Examples are syringomyelia, Arnold-Chiari malformation, and diastematomyelia. These conditions are often associated with spinal bifida.

Infection

Neurotropic viruses, e.g., herpes virus, poliovirus, and rabies may affect the spinal cord and/or the brain. The virus, however, cannot be identified in most cases.

Pyogenic infections of leptomeninges usually affect the sub-arachnoid space around the brain and the spinal cord. Epidural abscess may result from direct or haematogenous spread.

Tuberculous leptomeningitis produces spinal cord ischaemia by inflammatory arteritis. Tuberculous spinal osteitis (Pott's disease), with its associated psoas abscess and bony destruction, may cause cord compression or ischaemia.

Fungal infections (e.g., cryptococcosis) and parasitic infections (e.g., cysticercosis and hydatid disease) are rare in the spinal cord.

Neoplastic diseases

The lesion may be extradural, intradural-extramedullary, or intramedullary in location. The common benign lesions are neurofibroma and meningioma. The malignant lesions are ependymoma, astrocytoma, and carcinomatous meningeal infiltration. Related entities are paraneoplastic and irradiation myelopathy.

Diseases of the spine

- Spondylosis (*vide infra*)
- In longstanding rheumatoid arthritis, atlantoaxial or subaxial dislocation may cause cervical cord compression.

Vascular disorders

Diseases of the aorta, vertebral, intercostal, and radicular arteries may present as cord transection or anterior spinal artery syndrome. Acute spinal venous obstruction is rare and usually secondary to conditions such as tumour, septicaemia, and thrombotic diathesis; the prognosis is poor because of extensive haemorrhagic infarction. Vasculitis, e.g., in SLE, PAN, may give rise to acute spinal cord symptoms. AVM may either present with acute or chronic spinal cord features.

Demyelination

- Multiple sclerosis
- Post-infectious encephalomyelitis

Degenerative

- Spinocerebellar degeneration
- Idiopathic spastic paraparesis

Trauma (see Chapter 20)

Clinical picture and diagnosis

The clinical features depend on the pattern and level of the lesion (Figure 14.1).

Motor deficits

- UMN weakness below the lesion
- LMN weakness at the level of the lesion
- Mixed LMN and UMN weakness, e.g., upper limbs in cervical cord lesion
- Spinal shock stage: flaccid paralysis

Sensory disturbance

- Spinothalamic sensations: pain, temperature
- Posterior column sensations: vibration, joint position
- Sensory disturbance may present as a sensory level, glove and stocking distribution, segmental sensory loss, or dissociated sensory loss.
- Pain may arise from vertebral collapse or malignant infiltration of spinal root (radicular pain) or spinal cord.

Complete cord syndrome

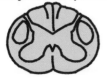

Central cord syndrome

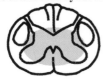

Brown-Séquard syndrome

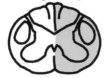

Anterior cord syndrome

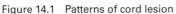

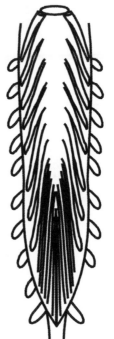

Conus ± cauda equina syndrome

Figure 14.1   Patterns of cord lesion
- Complete cord (acute or subacute): bilateral UMN paralysis and loss of all sensory modalities below lesion
- Brown-Séquard (hemicord): ipsilateral UMN weakness and loss of posterior column sensations, with contralateral loss of spinothalamic sensations below lesion
- Central cord: usually due to trauma of the cervical spinal cord. The damage to the central area results in bilateral upper limb weakness, with the lower limbs relatively less affected.
- Anterior cord: bilateral UMN paralysis and loss of spinothalamic sensations with sparing of posterior column sensations below lesion
- Conus medullaris/cauda equina: mixed UMN and LMN weakness and sensory deficits in the lower limbs, plus sphincter disturbances

Autonomic dysfunction

- Bladder: spastic or paralytic
- Bowel: incontinence ± constipation
- Sexual dysfunction

Differential diagnosis

- Guillain-Barré syndrome may present as a rapidly evolving tetraparesis. Distinguishing features include the presence of bulbar palsy, paresis of extraocular muscles and areflexia.
- Acute neuropathies: usually due to vasculitis or toxin.
- Myasthenia gravis: no sensory disturbance; ocular involvement is common.
- Acute occlusion of the terminal aorta may cause ischaemia of the cauda equina or proximal sciatic and femoral nerves. Rarely the spinal cord may be involved. Pale cold skin and loss of pulses in the lower limbs are clues to the diagnosis.
- Occlusion of anterior cerebral artery may cause bilateral infarction of the paracentral lobule, resulting in acute paraplegia, sphincter dysfunction, and loss of position sense with intact pain perception. The last feature distinguishes this entity from acute spinal cord syndrome.
- Falx meningioma with pressure effect on the leg areas of the cerebral cortex

Specific investigations

Investigations are guided by the clinical diagnosis, especially for the spinal level where the lesion is likely to be present.
- X-ray spine: vertebral lesions, e.g., collapse, spondylosis
- MRI spine: investigation of choice since the cord, subarachnoid space, and adjacent tissues can be clearly visualized. CT spine or myelogram may be indicated if MRI is not available.
- CSF analysis: useful in infection, demyelination, and neoplastic meningitis

NB: LP may cause further deterioration if there is cord compression.

SELECTED ENTITIES

Acute spinal cord compression

It is a neurological emergency caused by:
- Malignancy: carcinomatous metastasis, lymphoma, myeloma
- Infection: tuberculous or pyogenic abscess, vertebral collapse
- Epidural haematoma: spontaneous, traumatic
- Acute disc protrusion

Urgent MRI is indicated to confirm or exclude spinal cord compression.

High-dose IV steroids can be given prior to confirmation with neuroimaging. Upon confirmation, urgent neurosurgical decompression or radiotherapy should be arranged. Delay of treatment is associated with poor recovery of function.

Transverse myelitis

The causes include viral infection, SLE, post-infectious demyelination, NMOSD, and MS. Note any history of viral infection or vaccination and previous episodes of neurological deficits. Acute spinal cord compression must be excluded.

MRI is indicated to visualize the lesion and exclude cord compression.

CSF analysis commonly shows lymphocytosis, normal glucose, normal or slightly raised protein. Oligoclonal IgG indicates intrathecal synthesis of IgG; it is a non-specific finding although commonly present in demyelination.

Treatment depends on the underlying cause.

Degenerative disease of the spine

If the spinal canal is constitutionally narrow, degenerative tissues of the spine (e.g., osteophytes, discs, ossified posterior longitudinal ligament, hypertrophied ligamentum flava) are more likely to cause compression of the spinal cord or roots.

Cervical spondylotic myelopathy (CSM)

Cervical spondylosis as a radiological feature is very common, and CSM is the most common cause of cervical cord lesion in subjects over age 50.

Males are more affected than females. A history of neck injury, neck pain, and stiffness can be elicited in some patients. The symptomatology is that of a cervical cord lesion, with or without spinal root lesion.

The mechanisms by which cervical spondylosis brings about cord damage are complex. Compression due to acquired spondylotic changes on top of a constitutionally narrow canal (sagittal diameter < 10 mm) is the most important factor. In addition, dynamic factors, viz. friction with osteophytes, pressure from the ligamentum flava, vertebral subluxation, and hyperextension injury also play a part. These mechanisms lead to impairment of microcirculation at the arteriolar level resulting in ischaemic cord damage. The differential diagnosis is that of other cervical cord lesions, e.g., neurofibroma, syringomyelia. Motor neurone disease, at its early stage, may mimic CSM.

Cervical spine radiography provides information on the sagittal diameter of the spinal canal, the presence and degree of spondylotic tissues, and the presence of vertebral subluxation. MRI (Figure 14.2) shows the degree and site of spinal cord and root compression and is the investigation of choice. SEP study may document posterior column deficits and is helpful in monitoring progress.

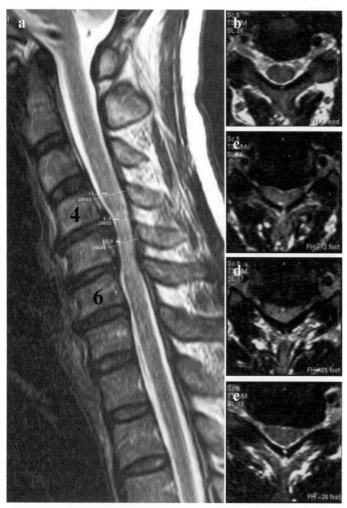

Figure 14.2   Sagittal (a) and axial (b to e) T$_2$ weighted MRI images of the cervical spine showing marked cervical spondylotic compression of the spinal cord at (c) C4/5 and (d) C5/6 levels but not at (b) C3/4 and (e) C6/7 levels.

Treatment is conservative for patients with mild symptoms and/ or a long history with little or no progression. However, surgery is indicated for patients with significant symptomatology or progression, and for those in whom conservative treatment has failed.

Cauda equina compression by lumbar prolapsed intervertebral disc (LPID)

LPID is common but in most cases, it either causes compression of a single spinal root (e.g., sciatica) or no neurological damage. Central protrusion of the disc into the spinal canal occurs uncommonly but may lead to acute or subacute cauda equina compression. It occurs more often at L4/5 and L5/S1 levels, hence the lowermost lumbar roots and sacral roots are affected.

The clinical picture is typical, and features include low back pain with or without radiation to both lower limbs; reduced sensation in the buttocks, perineum, and posterior thighs; absent ankle jerks; and sphincter disturbances with urinary retention, constipation and erectile dysfunction. Weakness in the lower limbs, especially of foot movements, may be present.

Diagnosis is made on clinical grounds and confirmed by MRI. Early diagnosis and prompt surgical decompression may partially or completely reverse the deficits.

Intermittent claudication of cauda equina

The underlying pathology is stenosis of the lumbar spinal canal, often due to spondylotic tissues superimposed on a constitutionally narrow canal.

The clinical features consist of weakness, reduced tendon reflexes, and sensory disturbance in the legs after walking a certain distance. At rest, these features may be absent. The differential diagnosis is peripheral vascular disease in which case the pulses in the legs are weak or absent.

X-ray of lumbar spine shows the degenerative bony changes and alignment. MRI confirms the diagnosis and provides information for surgical management.

Surgical decompression is indicated for patients with severe or progressive symptomatology.

Multiple sclerosis (see Chapter 9)

Syringomyelia

This is a classic example of an intramedullary lesion, with cavitation of the central part of the spinal cord, often extending vertically in the central grey matter over many segments. It presents with segmental sensory impairment of spinothalamic sensations due to disruption of decussating fibres at the anterior commissure. Extension of the syrinx to the anterior horns causes segmental amyotrophy, whereas extension to the posterior horns causes segmental loss of posterior column sensations. Functional disturbances of the legs and sphincters occur at a late stage.

Syringobulbia is due to extension of syrinx to the brainstem, resulting in lower cranial nerve palsy and disturbance of facial sensations.

About half of all idiopathic cervical syringomyelia cases are associated with type I Arnold-Chiari malformation in which the neck may be short and congenital abnormalities of the cervical spine and base of skull may be present. Secondary syringomyelia may complicate obstruction of the foramen magnum by localized arachnoiditis, cyst or tumour.

X-ray cervical spine and base of skull may show skeletal abnormalities. In MRI cervical spine (Figure 14.3), the location and extent of the syrinx, as well as cerebellar tonsillar herniation, can be visualized. MRI brain shows syringobulbia and other associated abnormalities.

Decompression of the syrinx is the treatment for symptomatic patients, particularly for those with Arnold-Chiari malformation.

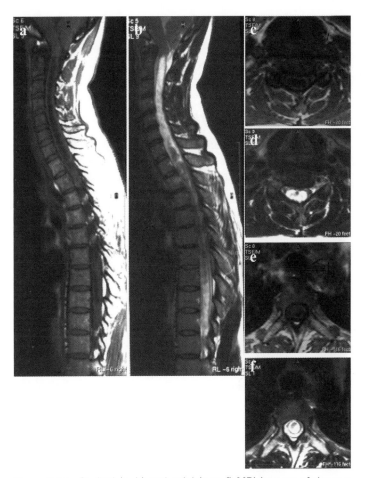

Figure 14.3 Sagittal (a, b) and axial (c to f) MRI images of the cervical and thoracic spine showing an expanded spinal cord due to a large syrinx which is hypointense on T_1 weighted (a, c, e) images and hyper-intense on T_2 weighted (b, d, f) images; (c) and (d) are at C4/5 level, and (e) and (f) at T3/4 levels. There is evidence of type I Arnold-Chiari malformation with cerebellar tonsillar herniation at the cervicomedullary junction in (a) and (b).

Spinocerebellar ataxia (SCA)

In most cases, including the SCA type 3, the inheritance is autosomal dominant. Sporadic cases are far less common. The symptoms start in the 30s or earlier. The progression is usually slow, and disability is moderate to severe. Degeneration of corticospinal and spinocerebellar tracts results in cerebellar ataxia and pyramidal signs. Associated features are uncommon and include peripheral neuropathy, optic neuropathy, cardiomyopathy, and cardiac arrhythmia. Cognition is intact. There is no curative treatment. Genetic diagnosis (including preimplantation) for the affected family is available.

Subacute combined degeneration of spinal cord

This is a classical and treatable condition due to vitamin B_{12} deficiency which may occur in pernicious anaemia, dietary insufficiency, and gastric or ileal resection. The pathological changes are degeneration of the lateral and posterior columns of the spinal cord, and to a lesser extent the brain and peripheral nerves. The patient presents with spastic tetraparesis, impaired posterior column sensations, peripheral neuropathy, and occasionally encephalopathy.

The diagnosis is made upon confirmation of vitamin B_{12} deficiency (e.g., megaloblastic anaemia, low serum B_{12}) and exclusion of other spinal cord lesions. The cause of vitamin B_{12} deficiency should also be elucidated.

Treatment is by parenteral vitamin B_{12} replacement. Hypokalaemia may develop during treatment. Early treatment confers a better chance of complete recovery.

Paraneoplastic myelopathy

This is not caused by spinal cord compression or invasion by carcinoma. The clinical syndrome is a rapidly developing non-inflammatory myelopathy with motor and sensory dysfunction.

Pathologically, there is necrosis of the tracts of the spinal cord without evidence of neoplasm. Anti-tumour antibody cross-reactive to the spinal cord has been proposed as the mechanism.

Irradiation myelopathy

The lesion evolves over a period of weeks and then becomes permanent. The total dose, fractionation, and size of radiated field are important factors. In general, fractionated irradiation up to a total dose of 3,500 rad is relatively safe. Irradiation induces obliterative endarteritis and thus ischaemic necrosis of the spinal cord tissues. The time interval between irradiation and the first spinal cord symptom varies, but usually ranges from 6–48 months. CSF is either normal or shows a slightly elevated protein level.

15 Peripheral Neuropathy

The peripheral nervous system includes the cranial nerves (except the optic nerve), the spinal nerve roots, the dorsal root ganglia, the peripheral nerve trunks, and the peripheral autonomic system.

The clinical patterns of neuropathies are:
- Polyneuropathies/polyradiculopathies
- Mononeuropathy
- Mononeuritis multiplex

The pathology is broadly classified as axonal degeneration, demyelination, and mixed. The clinical features are summarized in Table 15.1 and the common causes of polyneuropathies are listed in Table 15.2. However, it should be recognized that the cause may not be established in up to one-third of patients with chronic progressive neuropathies.

Differential diagnosis

Myopathy: Polymyositis without tenderness may mimic AIDP, but EMG features are diagnostic and CK is usually elevated.

Myasthenia gravis: It can be distinguished on clinical grounds, e.g., presence of fatiguability.

Eaton-Lambert syndrome: It may present with distal paraesthesia and hyporeflexia in addition to weakness; electrophysiology tests are diagnostic (facilitation of MAP after exercise).

Spinal muscular atrophy: It is difficult to clinically differentiate from motor neuropathies. NCS is helpful.

Tables 15.1 Clinical features of peripheral neuropathy

Motor	Negative motor symptoms: weakness, paralysis
	Positive motor symptoms: fasciculations, myokymia, muscle cramps
	Restless legs
	Neuromyotonia: persistent rhythmic motor unit activity up to 300 Hz
	Absent or reduced tendon reflexes: hallmark of peripheral neuropathy, often the first sign
Sensory	Negative sensory symptoms: small fibre vs large fibre sensory loss
	Positive sensory symptoms: paraesthesia, neuropathic pain, causalgia
	Painful legs and moving toes
	Intermittent symptoms: in carpal tunnel syndrome, meralgia paraesthetica
Autonomic	Postural hypotension, anhidrosis, incontinence, impotence
Others	Skeletal deformity: claw hand, pes cavus, kyphoscoliosis
	Trophic changes: disuse atrophy, trophic ulcers, osteoporosis, neuropathic joint
	Nerve thickening: in leprosy, acromegaly, HMSN, CIDP, neurofibromatosis

Table 15.2 Causes of polyneuropathy

Aetiology	Examples
Hereditary	HMSN
Infection	Leprosy, diphtheria
Toxic	Lead poisoning, n-hexane, vincristine, isoniazid
Metabolic	DM*, alcoholism*, uraemia*, vitamin B_{12} deficiency, amyloidosis, porphyria
Inflammatory	AIDP*, CIDP*
Paraneoplastic	Lymphoma, myeloma, carcinoma
Collagen vascular	SLE, rheumatoid arthritis
Degenerative	Dysautonomia

*Neuropathies commonly encountered in clinical practice.

Radiculopathies/plexopathies: Weakness and sensory loss in segmental distribution

Tabes dorsalis: Dissociated sensory loss with or without autonomic involvement; Charcot's joint

Myelopathy: Distal paraesthesia may precede long tract signs; early dorsal column deficits with posterior compression; tendon reflexes are either normal or increased.

Psychogenic weakness: Fluctuating and variable symptoms are common. The weakness often does not conform to neuroanatomical principles.

SELECTED ENTITIES

Hereditary neuropathies

- Hereditary motor sensory neuropathy (HMSN) or Charcot-Marie-Tooth disease
  - Type I (AD, hypertrophic form) is characterized by thickened nerves (50%), pes cavus, and inverted champagne bottle appearance of lower limbs. Hypertrophic changes (onion bulb) are characteristic, resulting from chronic demyelination and remyelination. NCV is markedly slow.
  - Type II (AD, neuronal form) is similar to Type I but is distinguished by a later onset of symptoms, relatively normal nerve conduction and absence of peripheral nerve thickening.
  - Type III (AR, hypertrophic neuropathy of childhood) is characterized by infantile onset, delayed motor development, severe sensory ataxia, skeletal deformities, marked NCV slowing, and confinement to wheelchair before age 20.
  - Type IV (AR) is milder than Type III with walking impairment developing in adolescence.
- Hereditary sensory autonomic neuropathy (HSAN), e.g., dysautonomia
- Neuropathy associated with spinocerebellar ataxia

- Hereditary neuropathies associated with specific metabolic defects, e.g., familial amyloid polyneuropathies, porphyria, abetalipoproteinaemia

Acute nerve injury

It is customary to classify nerve injuries into neuropraxia, axonotmesis, and neurotmesis with respect to the physical and functional state of the damaged nerve. NCS and EMG 2 weeks after injury are useful in differentiating these categories.

Neuropraxia

- Nerve dysfunction lasting several hours to 6 months
- Usually follows a blunt injury or compression
- Dysfunction attributed to focal demyelination, axonal membrane transport defect, mild ischaemia or haemorrhage
- Intact nerve axon with partial neurological deficits
- Recovery usually within 6 weeks but occasionally up to 6 months

Axonotmesis

- Axon disruption with intact epineurium
- No functional conduction but axonal regeneration will take place

Neurotmesis

- Complete interruption of the entire nerve with total nerve dysfunction
- Subsequent Wallerian degeneration and slow axonal regeneration (1 mm/day)
- Nerve graft or suture is often indicated to secure reunion and good functional recovery.
- Surgical exploration may be necessary to differentiate it from axonotmesis.

Brachial plexopathy

The brachial plexus is formed by the union of the ventral rami of spinal nerves C5-8 and T1 (C5+C6 form the upper trunk, C8+T1 form the lower trunk, and C7 becomes the middle trunk). The fibres are reassembled to form the lateral, posterior, and medial cords, from which the nerves supplying the upper limb are derived.

Traumatic

- May affect the whole, upper (Erb's palsy), or lower (Klumpke's palsy) plexus
- Stretch/traction, e.g., during birth, fall, general anaesthesia (the hypotonic arm being hyper-abducted)
- Compression, e.g., carrying heavy backpacks, axillary haematoma or aneurysm

Malignancy

- The Pancoast syndrome is due to carcinoma of the lung apex invading the lower trunk; coexisting Horner's syndrome is common.
- Lymph node or bone metastasis due to breast carcinoma infiltrating the brachial plexus

Radiation

- Radiation-induced fibrosis of the brachial plexus is dose-dependent (more likely if > 6,000 rads), which may occur 3 months to 20 years following irradiation.
- Upper trunk more often affected
- Differentiation from metastatic infiltration difficult and may require a combination of EMG, CT/MRI scanning of the plexus and isotope bone scan. Surgical exploration may be required to establish the diagnosis.
- No effective treatment; prognosis for neurological recovery poor

Thoracic outlet syndrome (TOS)

- The thoracic outlet comprises the first rib, apex of the lung, clavicle, brachial plexus, and subclavian artery and vein.
- TOS is due to stretching or compression of the lower trunk by an abnormal fibrous band, elongated transverse process of C7 vertebra or cervical rib, resulting in weakness and sensory deficits in the innervated territory.

Acute brachial plexus neuropathy (Brachial neuritis)

- The aetiology is often unknown, but triggering events include infection, immunization, pregnancy, irradiation, immunotherapy for malignancy, heroin abuse, trauma, and surgery.
- Characterized by severe pain radiating from shoulder to arm or neck, and lasting from a few hours to weeks. This is followed by flaccid paralysis of shoulder girdle or arm muscles (may be bilateral or unilateral, often partial and patchy), with or without sensory loss over the C5/6 distribution.
- The deltoid, serratus anterior, supraspinatus, and infraspinatus muscles are most commonly involved followed by the biceps and triceps. Muscle wasting is common.
- Treatment is mainly symptomatic, e.g., analgesics ± steroids for pain relief, physiotherapy to prevent frozen shoulder.
- The majority of patients recover by the end of second year; 5% of patients may have recurrence on the same or opposite side.

Lumbosacral plexopathy

The lumbosacral plexus is formed from the ventral rami of spinal nerves L1–S4. The femoral and obturator nerves arise from the lumbar roots. The sciatic nerve is derived from the L4–S2 roots.

Traumatic

- Fracture pelvis
- Gunshot injury

- Difficult labour causing compression of lumbosacral trunk (foot-drop and L5/S1 weakness pattern) in women
- Stretch injury in neonate following breech extraction

Malignancy

- The primary tumour often arises from the prostate, cervix, kidney, bladder, intestine, bone, and lymph nodes.
- It may be the earliest manifestation of malignancy.
- It is characterized by insidious onset of low-back or pelvic pain radiating to the lower limb followed by weakness and sensory loss.
- CT/MRI of lower abdomen and pelvis, neurophysiological studies, and isotope bone scan are helpful in establishing the diagnosis.

Radiation

- Onset 1 month to 30 years following irradiation to lumbar or pelvic region
- Begins with painless weakness in the legs (bilateral or asymmetrical) with or without numbness and paraesthesia
- Anterior horn cell damage and retroperitoneal fibrosis are possible mechanisms of injury.

Retroperitoneal lesion

- Psoas haematoma or abscess may produce mild or extensive lumbar plexopathy.
- The hip is usually kept in flexion posture since hip movement may increase pain.

Diabetic radiculoplexopathy (diabetic amyotrophy or lumbosacral plexopathy or Bruns-Garland syndrome)

- Occurs in poor glycaemic control or in mild stable DM; an ischaemic ± metabolic cause has been postulated.

- Onset may be insidious or acute; distribution can be bilateral or asymmetrical.
- Pain in the back, hips, and thighs is common with wasting and weakness involving hip girdles and thighs.
- Severity varies from mild to marked weakness but full recovery is possible.
- Imaging study (preferably MRI lumbar spine) to exclude compressive radiculopathy or cauda equina syndrome.

Nerve entrapment and pressure

Both nerve entrapment and pressure may result in mononeuropathy at specific sites (Table 15.3) where the nerve is confined to a narrow anatomical tunnel and hence susceptible to pressure from adjacent tissues, e.g., bony callus and fibrous band.

Table 15.3   Common sites of entrapment neuropathies

	Peripheral nerve	Site of compression
Upper limb	Median	Carpal tunnel (at wrist)
		Forearm (anterior interosseous nerve)
	Ulnar	Cubital tunnel (at elbow)
		Guyon's canal (at wrist)
	Radial	Axilla, spiral groove
Lower limb	Sciatic	Sciatic notch (piriformis syndrome)
	Lateral cutaneous nerve of thigh	Inguinal ligament (meralgia paraesthetica)
	Peroneal	Fibular neck
		Anterior compartment
	Posterior tibial	Medial malleolus (tarsal tunnel syndrome)

Median nerve

At wrist

- Carpal tunnel syndrome (CTS) is common.
- Often idiopathic, but may be associated with pregnancy, RA, DM, thyroid disease, acromegaly, and repetitive wrist movements .

- Due to pressure on the nerve from the thickened flexor retinaculum
- Usually affects women
- Early symptoms consist of bouts of pain and paraesthesia in the wrist and fingers and adjacent palm; occasionally these may spread to the arm and shoulder; nocturnal sleep disturbance is common.
- The signs include weakness and wasting of the abductor pollicis brevis, sensory deficits in the radial 3½ fingers, positive Tinel's sign or Phalen's sign.
- Differential diagnosis includes C6/7 radiculopathy, lower brachial plexopathy, and functional disorder.
- Diagnosis is confirmed by NCS/EMG.
- Conservative treatment for mild cases: wrist splint, local steroid injection. Surgical decompression for significant motor deficit or failed conservative treatment.

At forearm or above

- Anterior interosseous neuropathy leads to pure motor deficit with difficulty in pinching with the thumb and index finger.
- Causes: trauma (e.g., laceration in the forearm), unknown
- More proximal median neuropathy may result from damage following catheterization of the brachial artery, venepuncture or fracture of the humerus.

Ulnar nerve

At axilla

- Common causes: compression during coma, misuse of crutches, subclavian artery aneurysm or haematoma
- The median and radial nerves may be involved concomitantly.

At elbow

Structural lesion at the condylar groove or cubital tunnel
- Fractures, elbow joint deformities, cubitus valgus

- Pressure/trauma, e.g., leaning of elbow on hard surface, pressure injury during anaesthesia
- Soft tissue mass, e.g., ganglion, epidermoid cyst, lipoma
- Fibrous bands, supracondylar spurs, cubital tunnel syndrome

The clinical features include:
- Weakness and wasting of ulnar-innervated intrinsic hand muscles (claw hand)
- Sensory loss of ulnar distribution (ulnar 1½ fingers and adjacent palm)
- Tinel's sign at elbow
- Differential diagnosis includes lower brachial plexus lesions, C8/T1 radiculopathies, syringomyelia, and motor neurone disease.

At wrist

- Commonly due to trauma at the Guyon's canal
- Weakness of all ulnar-innervated intrinsic hand muscles together with sensory loss of the superficial terminal branch (sparing dorsal side); more distal lesions may spare the abductor digiti minimi.

Management

- Avoid further pressure or trauma
- Elbow padding in mild cases
- Surgical decompression, e.g., dividing aponeurosis of flexor carpi ulnaris, anterior transposition of ulnar nerve.

Radial nerve palsy

- Nerve compressed at the spiral groove or upper medial arm
- Often following deep sleep (e.g., drunkenness, anaesthesia)

- Signs include wrist or finger drop, weakness of brachioradialis and triceps (for more proximal lesion), and variable sensory loss along dorsolateral aspect of the hand and the first three digits. A lesion above the spiral groove produces sensory loss at the dorsolateral aspect of arm and forearm due to involvement of the posterior cutaneous nerve of the arm and forearm.
- Differential diagnosis: isolated posterior interosseous palsy, C7 radiculopathy

Common peroneal nerve

- Common causes: external compression (during anaesthesia, coma, sleep, plaster, braces, habitual leg crossing, prolonged squatting), direct trauma (fracture fibula), soft tissue mass (ganglion, Baker's cyst), tumour, fibular tunnel entrapment, and systemic disease (DM, leprosy)
- Results in weakness of dorsiflexion and eversion of the foot and extension of the toes (foot drop), and sensory loss over the anterolateral aspect of the lower leg and dorsum of the foot and toes
- Differential diagnosis: L5 radiculopathy, lesions of lumbosacral trunk, and sciatic neuropathy
- Management: surgical decompression for mass lesion, fracture or compartment syndrome, nerve repair for complete transaction, tendon transfer for permanent cases; foot-drop brace or light weight plastic orthosis for functional improvement

Diabetic neuropathies

Neuropathies are the most common complications of DM. About 8% of diabetics have neuropathy at the time of diagnosis and about 50% have neuropathy after 25 years. They can be broadly classified as focal and multifocal neuropathies, polyneuropathies, and diabetic amyotrophy (Table 15.4).

Table 15.4   Classification of diabetic neuropathies

Classification	Entities

Focal and multifocal neuropathies	Cranial mononeuropathies (e.g., III, IV, VI, VII)
	  – III: pupil sparing and usually recovers in months
	Limb mononeuropathy
	Truncal (thoracoabdominal) radiculopathy
	  – symmetrical (anterior wedge shape sensory loss)
	  – asymmetrical (subacute segmental, i.e., paraesthesia)
	Entrapment neuropathies
	Multiple mononeuropathies (mononeuritis multiplex)
	Symmetrical proximal motor neuropathy

Polyneuropathies	Distal symmetrical polyneuropathy
	  – mixed sensory-motor-autonomic neuropathy
	  – predominantly sensory neuropathy (pseudosyringomyelic or pseudotabetic)
	  – predominantly motor neuropathy
	  – predominantly autonomic neuropathy
	  – hyperglycaemic neuropathy (transient distal paraesthesia)

Diabetic amyotrophy (proximal asymmetrical motor neuropathy)	Severe pain in the hip and thigh and asymmetrical weakness and wasting of thigh muscles

Treatment

- Improve glycaemic control.
- Symptomatic treatment
  - Analgesics: NSAID, tramadol, paracetamol
  - AEDs: gabapentin, pregabalin, carbamazepine
  - Antidepressants: amitriptyline, venlafaxine, duloxetine
- Treatment of autonomic dysfunction
  - Postural hypotension: elastic stocking, increase salt intake, fludrocortisone
  - Delayed gastric emptying: metoclopramide, domperidone
  - Diarrhoea: tetracycline
  - Recurrent urinary tract infections: consult a urologist

- Skin care to avoid trophic ulcers and infection
- Pancreatic transplantation: may halt progression of neuropathy
- Rarely an inflammatory vasculopathy may produce a rapidly progressive peripheral neuropathy in diabetics; it may respond to plasmapheresis or IVIG.

Acute inflammatory demyelinating polyradiculoneuropathy (AIDP) or Guillain-Barrè syndrome (GBS)

AIDP is an acquired neuropathy of immunological pathogenesis. Two-thirds of cases are preceded by upper respiratory infection, immunization or gastroenteritis. Organisms of the antecedent infection may include HSV, CMV, EBV, HBV, mycoplasma or *Campylobacter jejuni*. It may be associated with lymphomas, collagen vascular disease or HIV carrier state. The mortality in modern ICU setting is between 1% and 5%.

Clinical features

- Generalized hypo-reflexia
- Symmetrical weakness from distal to proximal
- Respiratory failure in 10–20%
- Cranial nerves affected in 45–75% (VII in 50%)
- Mild sensory disturbance: paraesthesia, myalgia, back pain, impaired vibration or joint position sense
- Autonomic disturbance: labile BP, cardiac arrhythmias
- Raised ICP, papilloedema

Clinical variants of AIDP/GBS

- Miller-Fisher syndrome: triad of ophthalmoplegia, sensory ataxia, and areflexia; associated with anti-GQ_{1b} ganglioside antibody
- Polyneuritis cranialis: rapid onset of multiple cranial nerve palsies

- Acute pandysautonomia: rapid onset of sympathetic and para-sympathetic failure
- Axonal form of GBS: tetraplegia with bulbar and respiratory involvement

Complications

- Respiratory: insufficiency, hypostatic or aspiration pneumonia
- Urinary tract infection, bedsore
- DVT, pulmonary embolism
- Ileus
- Cardiac arrhythmias, sudden death
- Reactive depression

Investigations

- CSF analysis:
  - Protein-cell dissociation is characteristic, but about 10% of patients have normal protein especially during the first week of illness.
  - Mild pleocytosis may be present, but cells > 50/µl should raise the suspicion of Lyme disease or HIV infection.
- Neurophysiology tests:
  - Most cases have abnormal NCS indicating demyelination ± axonal degeneration.
  - Denervation changes occur at a later stage.

Supportive treatment

- Monitor FVC, ABG, blood pressure, and bulbar functions.
- Consider intubation if FVC deteriorating or below one litre (or 12 ml/kg), low PaO_2 or respiratory fatigue.
- Chest physiotherapy and breathing exercise
- Tracheostomy if prolonged ventilation is needed, especially in the presence of bulbar palsy
- Monitor and treat cardiac arrhythmias.
- Calcium heparin or LMWH to prevent DVT

- NSAID or narcotics for myalgia
- Regular turning if bedridden
- Artificial tears, taping of eyelids for corneal protection
- Physiotherapy and other measures to prevent contracture
- Psychological support

Specific treatment

Either intravenous immunoglobulins (IVIG) at 0.4 g/kg daily for 5 days or plasmapheresis (5 exchanges of 50 ml/kg/exchange) is effective treatment. If given early (< 2 weeks from onset), it will lead to earlier and smoother recovery, and pre-empt/shorten the use of ventilator. Indications include moderately severe disease and initially mild but deteriorating condition. However, some patients may not respond to one mode, in which case the other mode has to be used consecutively. Steroids confer no benefit.

Chronic inflammatory demyelinating polyradiculoneuropathy (CIDP)

CIDP is similar to AIDP in terms of clinical features, CSF findings, pathological abnormalities, NCS findings, and a suspected autoimmune aetiology. It is distinguished from AIDP by its more protracted course, relapses, lack of association with preceding infection, association with certain HLA (e.g., A1, B8, DR3, A3, DR2), and good response to steroid therapy.

Clinical features

- Symmetrical sensory and motor neuropathy
- No predilection for proximal lower limb muscles (in contrast to AIDP)
- Glove and stock distribution of numbness or tingling
- Postural tremor of upper limbs or pseudoathetosis
- Palpable or thickened peripheral nerves
- Papilloedema

- Bulbar or facial weakness
- Features of demyelination of the brainstem or spinal cord may be present.
- The clinical course may be progressive, relapse-remitting or monophasic.

Differential diagnosis

- Hereditary demyelinating neuropathies (characterized by uniform homogenous slowing of NCV and absence of conduction block)
- Acquired demyelinating neuropathies due to systemic disease, e.g., HIV-related, SLE, monoclonal gammopathy, multiple myeloma

Investigations

- NCS: multifocal conduction block, differential slowing of NCV in different nerve segments
- CSF study: protein-cell dissociation, positive oligoclonal band
- MRI brain and spinal cord may show evidence of central demyelination.
- Others: serum and urine immunoelectrophoresis, ESR, autoimmune screening

Nerve pathology

- Segmental demyelination by teased fibre technique
- Mononuclear cells infiltration
- Onion bulb formation
- IgM, IgG or complement deposits

Prognosis

- Most patients are ambulatory following treatment.

Management

- High-dose steroids; other immunosuppressives may be necessary.
- Plasmapheresis
- IVIG
- Lymphoid irradiation

Subacute inflammatory demyelinating polyneuropathy (SIDP)

This is characterized by a predominant motor demyelinating polyneuropathy which progresses within 4–8 weeks to peak deficits. It is characterized by its monophasic course, lack of respiratory or cranial nerve involvement, and steroid responsiveness. This recently recognized entity bridges the gap between AIDP and CIDP.

Paraneoplastic neuropathy

Subacute sensory neuronopathy (or carcinomatous sensory neuropathy)

The pathology consists of primary degeneration of dorsal root ganglion neurones with or without inflammation. It is probably immune-mediated due to anti-neuronal or anti-Hu antibodies, and is associated with carcinoma of lung (small cell), breast, ovary, gastrointestinal tract or Hodgkin's disease. Limbic encephalitis, myelitis or cerebellar degeneration may coexist. All sensory modalities are eventually affected. The response to treatment is poor.

Sensorimotor neuropathy

This is a symmetrical distal sensorimotor neuropathy progressing from the lower to upper limbs and is frequently preceded by significant weight loss.

The major pathological findings are axonal degeneration and loss of myelinated nerve fibres due to metabolic abnormality in axonal metabolism. This condition is associated with carcinoma of lung (small cell), breast, stomach, colon, pancreas, uterus, cervix, thyroid, and testis. The neuropathy may precede the diagnosis of malignancy.

Toxic neuropathies

- Most are distal axonopathies.
- Present with gradual onset of numbness and paraesthesia in the feet
- Onset concurrent with or shortly after exposure to toxin
- Generally improves after withdrawal of offending agent
- Common causes of toxic and drug-induced neuropathies (see Table 15.5)

Table 15.5   Some examples of toxic and drug-induced neuropathies

	Offending agents
Toxic neuropathies	Acrylamide, carbon disulphide, mercury, alcohol hexacarbons (e.g., n-hexane), arsenic, ethylene oxide, lead, organophosphates
Drug-induced neuropathies	Allopurinol, cis-platinum, metronidazole, disulfiram, hydralazine, amiodarone, chloroquine, colchicine, phenytoin, gold, isoniazid, amphetamines, dapsone, vinca alkaloids, heroin, lithium

Critical illness polyneuropathy

It is a diffuse polyneuropathy occurring in critically ill patients, often in the ICU setting. Tumour necrosis factor may be responsible for the pathogenesis. Patients usually present with difficulty in weaning off the ventilator. However, recovery is usually good for those who survive.

The disease predominantly affects the elderly with a mean onset at 28 days after the acute illness. Tetraparesis is common and sensory deficits minimal. NCS often shows features of axonal degeneration, and EMG may reveal widespread denervation changes. CSF analysis is within normal limits.

Management consists of ventilator support until there is adequate return of respiratory effort, and active physiotherapy to prevent bedsores and contractures.

Multifocal motor neuropathies

- A rare disorder which resembles MND
- Associated with high titres of anti-ganglioside (anti-GM_1) antibodies (see Table 15.6)
- Antibodies bind to motor end-plates or nodes of Ranvier
- They are usually IgM and polyclonal but may be monoclonal or IgG; possible association with plasma cell dyscrasia.
- Presents with progressive LMN limb weakness, which may be fulminant
- NCV slowing or multifocal conduction block; EMG shows denervation changes. Tongue fasciculations may be present.

Table 15.6   Conditions with positive anti-GM_1 antibodies titres

Anti-GM_1 antibodies titres	Conditions with positive titres
1:800	Normal subjects, multiple sclerosis, Alzheimer's disease, SLE
1:1600 to 1:3200	MND (IgG more likely), sensory neuropathy
1:6400	Motor neuropathy ± conduction block, UMN signs may be present

- Responds to plasmapheresis, IVIG infusion, or steroids plus cyclophosphamide
- May be difficult to differentiate from MND

Complex regional pain syndrome (reflex sympathetic dystrophy syndrome)

This is an uncommon condition and its pathogenesis is still debated. It follows an initiating noxious event (e.g., peripheral nerve injury, bone fracture). The major feature is continuing regional pain which is disproportionate to the inciting event. The other features, usually of distal predominance, include sensory dysfunction (hyperalgesia, allodynia), vasomotor dysfunction (changes of skin temperature or colour), abnormal sudomotor activity (sweating, oedema), trophic changes (of skin, hair, nail), decreased range of motion, and motor dysfunction (weakness, tremor, dystonia). Any condition which better explains the signs and symptoms must be excluded before the diagnosis is made. The course is often protracted. Prompt diagnosis and multidisciplinary treatment may yield better therapeutic results.

Anterior horn cell disease

Motor neurone disease (MND) / Amyotrophic lateral sclerosis (ALS)

- The worldwide incidence is 12 per 100,000 with a mean age of onset at 55.
- Common presenting symptoms include muscle weakness, fasciculation and wasting, dysphagia, dysarthria, walking difficulty, and dypsnoea.
- Objective sensory signs and visual abnormalities are characteristically absent.
- Investigations: NCS shows features of axonal degeneration but preserved conduction velocity. EMG shows fasciculations, marked denervation and re-innervation changes. Neuroimaging and blood tests are required to exclude other conditions, e.g., cervical myelopathy, foramen magnum lesions, lymphoproliferative disorder, hexosaminidase-A deficiency.
- For sporadic MND, four subtypes are recognized:

1. Classic amyotrophic lateral sclerosis: progressive UMN and LMN signs affecting at least two different regions of CNS (cerebrum, brainstem, spinal cord)
2. Primary lateral sclerosis: a pure spinal cord UMN syndrome with a slow rate of progression; diagnosis is by exclusion.
3. Progressive muscular atrophy: in about 10% of all adult-onset MND; signs and symptoms are restricted to LMN features with a slower rate of progression compared to ALS. The rapidly progressive course or involvement of the bulbar muscles would help to distinguish this condition from SMA.
4. Progressive bulbar or pseudobulbar palsy: weakness involving the bulbar region only. Important differential diagnosis includes myasthenia gravis, syringobulbia, and brainstem lesion.

- For familial MND, the mode of inheritance may be AD (superoxide dismutase (SOD1) missense mutations or non-SOD1 types), AR, or X-linked.
- Prognosis: median survival of MND between 2 and 5 years; 25% patients surviving for 5 years and 10% surviving for more than 10 years. Better prognosis for the non-classic MND sub-types.
- Treatment is mainly supportive and symptomatic, including mechanical ventilation for respiratory failure, gastrostomy for feeding, aids for communications, physiotherapy, antidepressants, anxiolytics, and antispasticity drugs.

Spinal muscular atrophy (SMA)

SMA constitutes an important differential diagnosis in patients presenting with muscle weakness or wasting. They are also known as hereditary motor neuronopathies. Clinically and genetically SMA are heterogeneous (Table 15.7). The muscle wasting is due to degeneration of anterior horn cells, which may be distal, proximal or bulbar. Early onset cases tend to develop scoliosis, lordosis, pes cavus or joint contractures. The diagnosis is aided by neurophysiology tests (normal NCS but denervation and reinnervation changes on EMG). Muscle biopsy may show neurogenic, myopathic or mixed changes. Differentiation from muscular dystrophies may sometimes be difficult. The aetiology of these conditions remains obscure. The prognosis is relatively good when compared with MND.

Table 15.7   Classification of spinal muscular atrophy

Types	Syndromes	Inheritance	Age at onset
Proximal			
Type I: Acute infantile	Werdnig-Hoffmann	AR	In utero–6m
Type II: Chronic childhood	Kugelberg-Welander	AR	3m–15y
Type III: Adult onset		AR	20–40y
Type IV: Juvenile onset		AD	6m–5y
Distal			
(Types. I–IV)	Spinal form of Charcot-Marie-Tooth disease	AD/AR	2–40y
Bulbospinal		XL	15–60y
Scapuloperoneal		AD/AR	2–70y
Facioscapulohumeral		AD	< 20y
Oculopharyngeal		AD	30–40y
Segmental		Sporadic	2–30y

16 Myopathy

Diseases of muscle usually result in proximal muscle weakness, leading to difficulty in climbing stairs, rising from a chair or combing hair. Waddling gait and lumbar lordosis are seen in patients with weakness of pelvic girdle muscles. Sensory signs are absent. Reflexes are usually preserved in early stages but reduced subsequently in proportion to the degree of weakness.

Definitions

Muscular dystrophy: A primary muscle disorder with a hereditary basis

Myotonia: repetitive firing of action potentials in skeletal muscle fibres in response to stimulation, manifesting as impaired relaxation and tonic spasms. Myotonia is typically elicited by percussion or voluntary contraction.

Myositis: Muscle disorders due to inflammatory changes that are usually immune-mediated

Metabolic myopathy: Impairment of synthesis of muscle ATP due to biochemical abnormalities

Periodic paralysis: Intermittent muscular weakness precipitated by metabolic or electrolyte abnormality

Congenital myopathy: Non-progressive muscle disorder of undetermined cause that usually occurs in children

Rhabdomyolysis: Muscle necrosis leading to myoglobinuria and markedly elevated muscle enzymes

Classification

Muscle disorders can be classified according to aetiology (Table 16.1).

Table 16.1   Classification of muscle disorders

Muscular dystrophies	Duchenne muscular dystrophy (XR) Becker dystrophy (XR) Facioscapulohumeral dystrophy (AD) Scapuloperoneal dystrophy (AD/XR) Oculopharyngeal dystrophy (AD) Limb girdle dystrophy (AD/AR)

Congenital	Myotonic disorders:
	  – Myotonic dystrophy (AD)
	  – Myotonia congenita (AD/AR)
	  – Paramyotonia congenita (AD)
	Non-myotonic disorders:
	  – Congenital hypotonia
	  – Prader-Willi syndrome
	  – Central core disease

Metabolic	Disorders of carbohydrate metabolism,
	  e.g., myophosphorylase deficiency
	Disorders of lipid metabolism, e.g., carnitine
	  palmityl transferase deficiency
	Abnormalities of mitochondrial function,
	  e.g., KSS

Endocrine	Hyperthyroidism, hypothyroidism Acromegaly Cushing's syndrome Hyperparathyroidism: primary, secondary Osteomalacia
Periodic paralysis	Hypokalaemic: familial, secondary Hyperkalaemic Normokalaemic
Inflammatory	Polymyositis/dermatomyositis: idiopathic, collagen diseases, neoplasm Inclusion body myositis Polymyalgia rheumatica Viral myositis, e.g., coxsackievirus Parasitic myositis, e.g., cysticercosis, trichinosis Drug-induced myositis, e.g., hydralazine

Investigations

Serum creatine kinase (CK)

Causes of marked elevation of CK (1000 to 10000 IU/l)

- Inflammatory myopathies
- Acute rhabdomyolysis
- Duchenne muscular dystrophy, Becker muscular dystrophy

Causes of moderate elevation of CK (200–1000 IU/l)

- Myopathies: most types
- SMA, MND
- Rigorous exercise
- Intramuscular injection especially of irritant drugs, e.g., chloroquine, diazepam, chlorpromazine
- After EMG or muscle biopsy
- Tonic-clonic seizures
- Acute myocardial infarction (isoenzyme CK-MB fraction > 12%)
- Drugs: statins, neuroleptics

NCS and EMG (see Chapter 2)

Muscle biopsy (see Chapter 2)

Specific biochemical screening

- Ischaemic lactate test if glycolytic enzyme deficiency is suspected
- Exercise lactate test if mitochondrial myopathy is suspected

Genetic study

- For inherited disorders such as muscular dystrophies and congenital myopathies

Treatment

General measures

- Physiotherapy, occupational therapy, aids, and social support are essential.
- Ventilatory support for patients with respiratory failure

Specific measures according to aetiology

- Genetic counselling for hereditary myopathies
- Immunosuppressive treatment for inflammatory myopathies
- Treat underlying metabolic abnormality for metabolic myopathies.
- Correct endocrine disturbance.

SELECTED ENTITIES

Duchenne muscular dystrophy (DMD)

The incidence is about 1 in 3,500 live births in Caucasian populations and the mode of inheritance is XR. The dystrophin gene is located at the short-arm of the X-chromosome. About 30–60% are deletions. This results in truncated dystrophin (a structural protein of the muscle sarcolemmal membrane) that is unstable, leading to active degeneration of muscles.

Typically, the male child develops symptoms at around 5 years old, with progressive weakness in the girdles and paraspinal muscles. Other features include pseudohypertrophy of calf muscles, cardiomyopathy, and intellectual subnormality. Patients usually become chair-bound in the second decade, and death due to respiratory or heart failure usually occurs in the second or third decade.

Treatment includes prevention and control of contractures, surgery for scoliosis, and ventilatory support. There is no evidence of benefit from steroid therapy. Early referral of the patient and his family for genetic counselling is essential. Carriers should be identified before they become pregnant. Prenatal diagnosis is available.

Becker muscular dystrophy

The mode of inheritance is XR. Dystrophin of abnormal molecular weight and quantity is produced. Compared with DMD, symptoms are milder and reach the same milestones about a decade later. Some patients survive to normal age with severe disability.

Myotonic dystrophy

This multisystem disease is of AD inheritance. It usually presents in young adulthood with varying severity and a slowly progressive course.

Clinical features

- Weakness and wasting of distal muscles, temporalis, sterno-mastoid, facial, and jaw muscles
- Myotonia of hand and tongue producing persistent handgrip and dysarthria respectively
- Dysphagia, ptosis, extraocular muscle weakness
- Frontal baldness, cataract, cardiac conduction defects
- Low intellect with or without dementia
- Obstructive sleep apnoea, pulmonary hypoventilation
- Endocrine dysfunction: hypothyroidism, DM, gonadal atrophy, and impotence
- Skull hyperostosis, small pituitary fossa
- Malignant hyperpyrexia

Management

- Muscle biopsy is not necessary because the clinical picture and EMG findings are diagnostic.
- Referral for genetic counselling
- Myotonia is often mild and does not require specific treatment.

Non-dystrophic myotonic syndromes

The clinical features of myotonia congenita (AD or AR inheritance) and paramyotonia congenita (AD inheritance) are listed in Table 16.2.

Table 16.2 Differentiating features between myotonia congenita and paramyotonia congenita

Myotonia congenita	Paramyotonia congenita
Present in infancy or childhood	Present in infancy
AD (Thomsen) or AR (Becker)	AD (Eulenburg)
Generalized myotonia	Attacks of myotonia
Worse in cold	Worse in cold and if hyperkalaemic
Relieved by warmth/exercise	Relieved by hypokalaemia
Minimal weakness	Flaccid weakness

An inherited abnormality of voltage-gated chloride channel of skeletal muscle (point mutations on chromosome 7q35) is present in myotonia congenita. The voltage-gated chloride channel helps in repolarization, and reduced chloride conductance leads to membrane hyperexcitability.

Voltage-gated sodium channels are crucial in the generation and propagation of muscle action potentials. In paramyotonia congenita, there is mutation of the gene encoding the sodium channel in chromosome 17q23. When muscle fibres are cooled to 27°C or below, sustained inward sodium current occurs, leading to membrane depolarization. The small but sustained depolarization leads to membrane hyperexcitability, muscle stiffness, and persistent contraction.

Treatment

Drug therapy (e.g., procainamide, phenytoin, disopyramide, nifedipine, quinine sulphate) is effective in relieving the symptoms. Avoid β-blockers and depolarizing muscle relaxants.

Mitochondrial encephalomyopathy

Three major syndromes are recognized: Kearn-Sayre syndrome (KSS); myoclonus epilepsy with ragged red fibres (MERRF); and mitochondrial encephalomyopathy, lactic acidosis, and stroke-like episodes (MELAS). Their clinical features are summarized in Table 16.3. The disease can be transmitted via maternal mitochondrial DNA. Muscle biopsy is necessary for diagnosis. Treatment is supportive.

Table 16.3   Clinical features of mitochondrial encephalomyopathy

Features	KSS	MERRF	MELAS
Ophthalmoplegia	+	−	−
Retinal degeneration	+	−	−
Heart block	+	−	−
Myoclonus	−	+	−
Ataxia	+	+	−
Seizures	−	+	+
Dementia	+	+	+
Short stature	+	+	+
Hemiparesis	−	−	+
Sensorineural deafness	+	+	+
Family history	−	+	+
Lactic acidosis	+	+	+
Raised CSF protein	+	−	−

+ = present; − = absent

Acid maltase deficiency

- AR inheritance
- Enzyme deficiency results in impaired lysosomal conversion of glycogen to glucose.
- In early onset form: death at infancy
- In adult onset form: slowly progressive weakness of proximal limb and respiratory muscles
- Respiratory failure may be the presenting symptom.

- CK is slightly elevated with non-specific changes on EMG and muscle biopsy.
- Diagnosis is based on assay of muscle enzymes or cultured skin fibroblasts.

Familial hypokalaemic periodic paralysis

- AD inheritance with variable penetrance in females; sporadic cases more common in males
- Most common form of inherited periodic paralysis
- Mutation in the α-subunit of skeletal muscle dihydropyridine-sensitive calcium channel gene in chromosome 1q32; mechanism unknown
- Male to female = 3 to 1; onset usually in the second decade
- Proximal muscle weakness > distal > respiratory weakness
- Paralysis is precipitated by heavy exercise, carbohydrate load, or hyperinsulinaemia, and commonly occurs after sleep.
- Muscle biopsy is usually normal or shows mild myopathic changes with vacuolation.
- Replacement of potassium for acute attacks and acetazolamide for prophylaxis are effective treatments.

Secondary hypokalaemic periodic paralysis

- High incidence in Asian populations; sporadic; male > female
- Associated with thyrotoxicosis, diuretics abuse, diuresis after alcohol binge
- Treatment is similar to the familial cases, but underlying causes should also be corrected. For patients with thyrotoxicosis, standard treatment applies.

Familial hyperkalaemic periodic paralysis (Gamstorp's disease)

- Rare, AD inheritance
- Episodic of muscle weakness and paralysis after exercise since infancy or childhood; inducible by potassium salts; recovery hastened by exercise

- Permanent weakness and proximal muscle wasting may develop from repeated attacks.
- Attacks diminish or cease in late adolescence or adulthood when the patient becomes more sedentary.
- Elevated serum potassium; myotonic symptoms common
- Point mutations in the human skeletal muscle sodium channel gene
- A persistently activated sodium current is found at very negative membrane potentials in biopsied muscle fibres. The depolarized muscles are inexcitable because of inactivation of sodium channels.
- Provocative test with oral potassium chloride under monitoring
- Same treatment as for paramyotonia congenita

Malignant hyperthermia

- Potentially lethal pharmacogenetic skeletal muscle disorder; AR inheritance much more common than AD; incomplete penetrance with variable expressivity; mortality 10–15%
- Estimated incidence 1 per 50,000–150,000 anaesthetic exposures; 50% with prior anaesthesia
- Symptoms manifest within minutes to hours following exposure to inhalational anaesthetic agents (e.g., halothane, enflurane, isoflurane), depolarizing muscle relaxants (e.g., succinylcholine, decamethonium, D-tubocurarine), or large volume of amide local anaesthetics (e.g., lidocaine, mepivacaine).
- Hyperthermia, rigidity, metabolic and respiratory acidosis, hyperkalaemia, rhabdomyolysis
- Variable severity
- Other features: tachycardia, cardiac arrhythmia, hypertension, hypotension, angina, vascular spasm with cyanosis, cardiac arrest
- Very high CK level, hypercalcaemia, DIC
- Pathogenic mechanisms: abrupt increase in intracellular calcium ion concentration in skeletal muscles due to abnormal accumulation of calcium ion by sarcoplasmic reticulum
- Mutations in the ryanodine receptor in chromosome 19q12–13.2; gene product functions as calcium release channel of the sarcoplasmic reticulum

- Some families have mutated $\alpha2/\delta$-subunits of the dihydropyridine-sensitive calcium channel in chromosome 7q.
- Principles of therapy: discontinuation of anaesthesia, IV dantrolene (1–4 mg/kg), body cooling, hydration, sodium bicarbonate infusion, mechanical ventilation, corticosteroids, and other supportive treatment
- Avoid general anaesthesia in susceptible individuals and family members; *in vitro* test of susceptibility using halothane and caffeine muscle contraction tests. Monitoring of end-tidal CO_2 level during anaesthesia facilitates early detection.

Neuroleptic malignant syndrome (NMS)

- Potentially lethal idiosyncratic reaction to neuroleptic treatment: within 2 weeks of initiation or increasing dosage; mortality about 5%
- Similar syndrome seen following dopamine-depleting medications or discontinuation of dopaminergic anti-parkinsonian therapy
- Estimated incidence 0.5–1.5%
- Clinical triad of fever, rigidity, and altered mentation (confusion to coma)
- A spectrum of severity
- Autonomic disturbance: tachycardia, excessive sweating, labile BP
- Other parkinsonian and extrapyramidal features: resting tremor, bradykinesia, dystonia, chorea
- Other neurological features: dysphagia, dysarthria, mutism
- Serious complications: rhabdomyolysis, myocardial infarction, cardiac arrest, persistent neurological deficit
- Laboratory findings: high CK, leukocytosis
- Symptoms intensify rapidly over next 24–72 hours; usually subside in 5–20 days following discontinuation of neuroleptic treatment
- Pathogenic mechanisms: mainly central dopaminergic blockage
  - striatum: generating shivering thermogenesis
  - diencephalons: cellular thermogenesis from sympathetic hyperactivity

- – hypothalamus: impaired heat dissipation from altered vaso-motor thermoregulatory control
- – muscles: possible direct action of neuroleptics on muscle contraction
- Principles of therapy: prompt recognition; discontinuation of neuroleptic treatment; body cooling; hydration; oral or naso-gastric central dopaminergic drugs (bromocriptine, levodopa, amantadine); IV dantrolene; consider pancuronium; other supportive treatments
- Recurrence of NMS may occur in 20% of patients following re-introduction of neuroleptics. Atypical neuroleptics (olanzap-ine, quetiapine, risperidone) are preferred.

Myoglobinuric myopathies or rhabdomyolysis

- The aetiology is listed in Table 16.4.
- Diagnosed by positive urine reaction with benzidine if haema-turia or haemoglobinuria is absent
- CK is invariably elevated, usually above 1000 IU/l.
- Acute renal failure may develop as a result of acute tubular necrosis.

Table 16.4   Aetiology of myoglobinuric myopathies

Enzyme deficiency, e.g., myophosphorylase deficiency, phosphofructokinase deficiency, carnitine palmityl transferase deficiency
Neuroleptic malignant syndrome
Malignant hyperthermia
Status epilepticus
Excessive exercise
Muscle ischaemia, e.g., severe burn, crush injury, sickle cell crisis
Alcohol
Drug-induced
Inflammatory myopathies
Snake bite

- Ensure adequate hydration; forced diuresis using mannitol or loop diuretics may be necessary in severe cases.

Polymyositis and dermatomyositis

It is an autoimmune disorder affecting voluntary muscles in all age groups. Associated skin involvement (or dermatomyositis) occurs in 30% of cases. Collagen vascular disease or malignancy (e.g., carcinoma of bronchus, NPC) is present in 25% of cases.

Clinical features

- Onset may be acute, subacute or insidious.
- Diffuse muscle weakness with symmetrical and proximal distribution
- Distal, bulbar, and respiratory muscles are rarely involved, and ocular muscles are spared.
- Painful myopathy in the acute form, and wasting ± contractures in the chronic form
- Characteristic violaceous (heliotrope) rash around the eyes, cheeks, forehead, upper trunk, or extensor surface of the limbs. Induration and subcutaneous periorbital oedema may be present.
- Raynaud's phenomenon, arthralgia, pulmonary fibrosis and myocarditis are rare.

Investigations

ESR and CK are markedly elevated but may be normal in the chronic or quiescent phase. Myoglobinuria may be present in severe cases. EMG often shows myopathic potentials with fibrillations, and muscle biopsy characteristically shows necrosis and chronic inflammatory cells with perivascular cuffing. Underlying malignancy and associated collagen vascular disease should be searched for. MRI of muscles is useful in the diagnosis and management of inflammatory myopathies. It helps to confirm the diagnosis and selection of biopsy site to reduce the false-negative rate. MRI can also identify patients with complete fatty replacement of the muscles for whom continued immunosuppressive therapy is no longer indicated.

The differential diagnosis includes parasitic myositis, trichinosis, and inclusion body myositis.

Management

Prednisolone (1 mg/kg) daily is given until there is clinical improvement. Then taper to the minimum effective dose and switch to alternate day regime. Withdraw steroids if the disease is in remission. Steroid-sparing immunosuppressive agents are often given concomitantly and first-line immunosuppressive drugs include methotrexate or azathioprine. In patients who do not respond to steroid or the first-line drugs, cyclosporine, tacrolimus, IVIG, plasmapheresis, cyclophosphamide, rituximab, thymectomy, total body irradiation have been used alone or in various combinations with varying success. Muscle strength (documented with dynamometer), walking time over a standard distance, ESR, CK level, and MRI are useful parameters for monitoring clinical progress and disease activity.

Viral myositis

- Pain and tenderness are prominent in viral myositis and may be out of proportion to weakness.
- Recovery is usually within weeks.
- CK may be elevated, and rhabdomyolysis may rarely occur.
- Bornholm disease is caused by coxsackievirus type B.
- Post-viral fatigue syndrome is a complication.

Endocrine myopathies

Hyperthyroidism may be associated with proximal myopathy, periodic paralysis, and dysthyroid eye disease. CK is normal, but EMG shows myopathic features.

Hypothyroidism may produce muscle cramps, slowing of reflexes, pseudohypertrophy, myxoedema, and rarely weakness and raised CK. In acute transient hypothyroidism, severe muscle pain, stiffness, marked elevation of CK, and myopathic changes may occur.

Acromegaly may cause muscle hypertrophy, wasting, weakness, and raised CK.

Cushing's syndrome commonly produces proximal myopathy affecting the lower limbs with normal CK.

17 Systemic Disease and Neurotoxicity

SYSTEMIC DISEASE

Systemic disorders can affect the nervous system through different mechanisms, e.g., hypoxia, decreased perfusion, embolism, and autoimmunity. It is important to distinguish the primary neurological complications associated with the systemic disorder from its secondary complications (arising from therapy or other causes) because the management differs. This section covers the more common systemic disorders with neurological manifestations.

Cardiovascular disorders

Neurological complications are common in cardiac disorders, and include:

- Syncope: may result from transient global ischaemia caused by hypotension, cardiac arrhythmias or outflow obstruction (e.g., hypertrophic obstructive cardiomyopathy). There may be premonitory symptoms, e.g., visual disturbances, paraesthesia, and dizziness. It must be differentiated from epileptic seizures (see Table 7.2).
- Cardiogenic embolism to the brain (see Chapter 6)
- Cerebral hypoxia (see Chapter 12)

Postural hypotension

- Clinical features are due to cerebral hypoperfusion and include dizziness, visual disturbance (e.g., blurred or tunnel vision), syncope, and drop attacks. The symptoms may occur when rising from a lying position or during Valsalva manoeuvre (e.g., straining).

- Causes:
  - Vasovagal syndrome. Most common form; associated with a rapid drop in heart rate and blood pressure
  - Cardiovascular disorders, e.g., arrhythmias, outflow obstruction, cardiac failure
  - Primary autonomic dysfunction, e.g., in neurodegenerative disorders
  - Secondary autonomic dysfunction, e.g., in diabetes mellitus
  - Alcohol and hypotensive drugs
- Investigations include monitoring of BP and ECG in lying and standing positions, Holter monitoring of cardiac rhythm, tilt-table test, and echocardiogram.
- Avoid sudden changes in posture, alcohol, and hypotensive drugs. Elastic stockings, abdominal corsets, increase in salt intake, and fludrocortisone may help.

Infective endocarditis

- Historically linked to chronic rheumatic and congenital heart disorders, but recent increase in incidence associated with prosthetic valves and IV drug abuse
- The infected emboli may cause cerebral infarction, microabscesses, and meningoencephalitis, and may present as focal deficits, epileptic seizures or impaired consciousness. The microemboli may give rise to splinter haemorrhages in nails (of fingers or toes) and Roth spots in fundi. Rupture of mycotic aneurysms can lead to SAH and ICH, and may occur after apparent cure of the endocarditis. ICH may also develop from septic arteritis or from haemorrhagic transformation of cerebral infarcts.
- Causative organisms include:
  - *Strept. pneumoniae, Staph. aureus*, and *Staph. epidermidis* in patients with prosthetic valves or IV drug addicts
  - Gram-negative bacteria, e.g., Pseudomonas, Haemophilus, Bacteroides, *E. coli*, Proteus species
  - Fungal, e.g., Candida and Aspergillus species, especially in immunocompromised patients or drug addicts

- Investigations include repeat blood cultures, ECG, echocardiogram, and CT/MRI brain. In suspected mycotic aneurysms, cerebral angiography must be performed, especially if anticoagulant is required, e.g., in patients with prosthetic valves.
- Antimicrobial therapy is the mainstay of treatment. Neurological manifestations usually respond to treatment. Resection of mycotic aneurysm may be considered if long-term anticoagulation is required.

Respiratory disorders

- Chronic pulmonary failure results in chronic hypoxia and hypercapnia and may manifest with neurological symptoms, e.g., headache, confusion, postural or flap tremor, myoclonus.
- Hypercapnia may cause cerebral vasodilatation, raised ICP with papilloedema.
- Hyperventilation may occur voluntarily or with metabolic acidosis (e.g., diabetic coma, drug-induced toxicity), resulting in hypocapnia, which in turn leads to cerebral vasoconstriction with dizziness, paraesthesia, visual disturbance, headache, and carpopedal spasms.

Acute mountain sickness (see Chapter 5)

Sleep apnoea

This condition is associated with prolonged and frequent apnoea, causing repeated reduction in blood oxygen saturation. Chronic sleep apnoea with hypoxia can cause secondary polycythaemia, cardiac arrhythmias, and pulmonary vasoconstriction. In more severe cases, pulmonary hypertension and cor pulmonale may develop.

Sleep apnoea can be:

- Obstructive sleep apnoea (OSA), which is more common. Airflow is obstructed in the upper airway, and diaphragmatic and chest wall movements are normal. These patients are in general obese with a short and thick neck. Symptoms include chronic snoring between apnoeic periods, restless sleep with frequent arousals, daytime sleepiness and poor concentration, and are worsened with alcohol, sedatives, and respiratory infections. Other causes include acromegaly, achondroplasia, and rarely multisystem atrophy. In children, OSA may be due to large tonsils.

- Neurogenic sleep apnoea presents with insomnia with absence of snoring and restless sleep. The lack of airflow is due to hypoventilation, and may be due to failure of central respiratory motor output or loss of chemoreceptor control. It may occur in disease in the brainstem (e.g., encephalitis, tumour, syringobulbia, stroke) or upper cervical spinal cord (e.g., trauma).

In certain diseases (e.g., myotonic dystrophy), sleep apnoea is a mix of both types.

Investigations include pulse oximetry, video recordings, ECG, and polysomnography during sleep. Specialist assessment of the upper respiratory tract may be indicated. There is no single treatment modality. Patients should exercise and reduce weight, and stop alcohol, smoking, and sedatives intake. Nasal continuous positive airway pressure (CPAP) is effective but long-term compliance may be poor because of rhinitis, nasal discomfort, conjunctivitis, and mask intolerance. Palatopharyngoplasty may be considered.

Connective tissue and related vasculitic disorders

Neurological complications may result from the production of autoantibodies and proinflammatory cytokines, microangiopathy, microinfarction, and demyelination.

Systemic lupus erythematosus (SLE)

Neuropsychiatric features may occur during the active or remission phase. They include:
- Episodic mood and psychotic disorders are common, and should be distinguished from sepsis or drug-induced mental changes. CSF IgM, IgA and IgG tend to be increased in SLE-induced

psychosis, unlike steroid-induced psychosis. The latter usually develops between 5 and 14 days after starting therapy, and is dose-dependent.

- Seizures may be associated with microinfarcts, metabolic disturbance and sepsis.
- Focal deficits may result from strokes (TIA, cerebral infarction, cerebral venous thrombosis) and transverse myelitis. Strokes may develop from valvular disease, thrombosis associated with antiphospholipid antibodies, and cerebral vasculitis.
- Headache is common and may be due to aseptic meningitis.
- Chorea, cognitive dysfunction, delirium
- Peripheral nervous system complications are less common, and usually presents as a sensorimotor polyneuropathy, Guillain-Barré syndrome, mononeuropathy and mononeuritis multiplex (cranial and peripheral), plexopathy or autonomic neuropathy.
- Secondary neurological complications from uraemia, hypertension, sepsis, and coagulopathy

The diagnosis of SLE-induced complications is based on clinical assessments and response to therapy. Serological and electrophysiological tests can help. MRI brain may show multiple focal lesions in the periventricular and subcortical white matter, cortical atrophy and diffuse white matter infarction.

Treatment includes:

- Symptomatic treatment, e.g., anticonvulsant, antipsychotic, antidepressant, antiplatelet, analgesic therapies
- Immunosuppressive treatment, e.g., corticosteroids, cyclophosphamide
- Dehydroepiandrosterone may help reduce disease activity and neurological complications.

Antiphospholipid antibody syndromes

Antiphospholipid antibodies (lupus anticoagulant and anticardiolipin antibodies) may be found in SLE and other connective tissue disorders. Apart from recurrent abortion, presence of these antibodies is associated with a (paradoxical) tendency to thrombosis, resulting in cerebral arterial or venous thrombosis.

Rheumatoid disease

Involvement of the central nervous system is uncommon. Peripheral neurological complications are more often encountered and include:

- Peripheral nerve involvement. Mild sensory neuropathy presents with symmetrical distal sensory deficit of glove and stocking distribution, with little or no weakness. Severe sensorimotor neuropathy often presents as acute mononeuritis multiplex, and is associated with vasculitis, destructive nodular rheumatoid arthritis, and widespread systemic vasculitic involvement.
- Entrapment neuropathy is common.
- Muscle atrophy may be due to neuropathy or disuse atrophy, because of joint destruction and contractures.
- Atlanto-axial subluxation at the cervical spine may cause myelopathy, headache, and pose a risk during endotracheal intubation. Avoid hyperextending the neck. Surgical fixation of the subluxation is usually not necessary.

Treatment includes NSAIDs, corticosteroids (intra-articular or systemic) and disease-modifying therapy (e.g., chloroquine, gold, penicillamine, methotrexate, azathioprine, mycophenolate, cyclophosphamide). Newer forms of disease-modifying therapies include anti-tumour necrosis factor (e.g., infliximab) and blockade of interleukin-6 signalling (e.g., tocilizumab). Gold and chloroquine may cause peripheral neuropathy. Penicillamine may cause myositis and myasthenic syndrome.

Behçet's disease

Apart from oral and genitourinary ulcers, relapsing uveitis and optic atrophy may develop. Neurological complications include focal or multifocal brainstem and spinal cord deficits resembling minor ischaemic strokes, aseptic meningitis and meningoencephalitis. CSF analysis may show mild pleocytosis with raised protein content. NSAIDs and corticosteroids are useful. Other immunomodulating agents include thalidomide, cyclophosphamide, interferon (α and γ), anti-tumour necrosis factor α (e.g., infliximab).

Sjögren's syndrome

Polyneuropathy is a relatively common manifestation, caused by small vessel vasculitis. Uncommon neurological complications include psychosis, cognitive deficits, migraine, transverse myelitis, and meningoencephalitis.

Systemic sclerosis (scleroderma)

The neurological complications usually present as a distal sensorimotor polyneuropathy or entrapment mononeuropathy. Myopathy and myositis may also develop.

Vasculitis and related syndromes

These include polyarteritis nodosa, Wegener's granulomatosis, Churg-Strauss syndrome and giant cell arteritis, and are caused by inflammation of the arteries and arterioles. Complications may develop from hypertension, and renal, cardiac, pulmonary, gastrointestinal, and skin involvement. The illness is preceded by prodromal symptoms, e.g., general malaise, weight loss, fever, myalgia, arthralgia.

Polyarteritis nodosa

May be complicated by:
- Peripheral neuropathy, which is common
- CNS involvement, which usually occurs later, manifesting as cognitive deficits, behavioural change, and acute confusion.
- Headache, which is common and may be due to aseptic meningitis
- Cerebral infarction or haemorrhage
- Episcleritis, anterior uveitis, retinal vasculitis

Wegener's granulomatosis and Churg-Strauss syndrome

In the former, involvement of the upper and lower respiratory tract and kidneys is prominent. In the latter, asthma (accompanied by allergic rhinitis) and eosinophilia are present. In both conditions, mononeuritis multiplex, multiple cranial nerve palsies and cerebral infarction may occur.

Giant cell (temporal or cranial) arteritis

This commonly occurs in the elderly, and is characterized by fever and severe pain and tenderness over the temporal scalp. Blindness may occur with ophthalmic artery occlusion. The ESR is markedly raised and neutrophilia present. Biopsy or arteriogram of the affected artery may be required for diagnosis. Corticosteroids and immunosuppressants are the mainstay of treatment.

Metabolic syndromes

Neurological disturbance may arise as a result of electrolyte disturbances, indirect hormonal effects, and direct metabolic effects on the nervous system.

Diabetes mellitus

This is the most common cause of polyneuropathy (see Table 15.2), and is a risk factor for strokes. Hypoglycaemia and hyperglycaemia can cause an acute encephalopathy presenting with confusion, stupor and life-threatening coma.

Pituitary tumour

Pituitary tumours typically cause bitemporal hemianopia due to compression of the optic chiasma, and optic atrophy may ensue. Growth hormone-secreting pituitary tumours may result in acromegaly, proximal myopathy, and carpal tunnel syndrome. In Cushing's syndrome, proximal muscle weakness, agitation, depression, psychoses, and stroke may develop.

Diabetes insipidus

This may result from hypothalamic or pituitary disorders. Transitory neurogenic diabetes insipidus often complicates head injuries or neurosurgical procedures, and may cause encephalopathy. It responds to DDAVP.

Hyperthyroidism

Hyperthyroidism can cause restlessness, headaches, and insomnia. Ophthalmic Graves' disease, which may occur in a euthyroid subject, is characterized by exophthalmos and ophthalmoplegia resulted from orbital oedema and inflammatory infiltrate.

Hypothyroidism

Hypothyroidism causes apathy, depression, cerebellar ataxia, hoarseness of voice, and in severe cases, myopathy and encephalopathy.

Electrolyte disturbances

Hypernatraemia and hyponatraemia

Abnormal serum sodium concentration may cause encephalopathy and coma. Seizures and myoclonus are common and may not respond to anticonvulsant therapy unless the sodium concentration is corrected. Hypernatraemia is caused by dehydration, diabetes insipidus, and overcorrection with IV saline. Hyponatraemia occurs in SIADH, iatrogenic water intoxication, and adrenocortical insufficiency. Rapid correction may result in central pontine myelinolysis.

Hypokalaemia

Hypokalaemia may cause marked muscle weakness, and in severe cases, rhabdomyolysis.

Hypercalcaemia and hypocalcaemia

Hypercalcaemia may present with encephalopathy characterized by apathy, agitation, and altered consciousness, and occurs in metastatic disease, myeloma, and hyperparathyroidism.

Hypocalcaemia may manifest with paraesthesia, muscle cramps, and tetany. In severe cases, epileptic seizures and encephalopathy may develop.

Neoplastic disorders

Neurological symptoms may be caused by direct invasion of the primary tumour, its metastatic and non-metastatic complications. These effects should be differentiated from iatrogenic complications, e.g., corticosteroids, chemotherapy, radiotherapy, opiates, sedatives. The common manifestations include headache, confusional state, epileptic seizures, neuropathic pain, and limb weakness.

Paraneoplastic syndromes of the nervous system

In paraneoplastic neurological disorders, an immunological response is triggered against an antigen expressed by the tumour cells. This anti-tumour immune response leads to damage of the nervous system when it targets the same antigen or a similar antigen which is expressed by cells of the nervous system. These onconeural antigens can be from membrane or intracellular proteins expressed in neurons, glia cells, peripheral nerves, neuromuscular junction, and muscle. Autoantibodies against these onconeural antigens may be detectable in serum and/or CSF of some patients, and hence facilitate the diagnosis of paraneoplastic neurological disorders. These antibodies include:

- anti-Hu antibodies (ANNA-1) in small cell lung carcinoma causing encephalomyelitis
- anti-Yo (PCA-1) and anti-Ri antibodies (ANNA-2) in gynaecological and breast cancers causing cerebellar degeneration

Paraneoplastic neurological disorders include:
- encephalitis: NMDAR, limbic, brainstem
- cerebellar ataxia
- opsoclonus-myoclonus
- myelitis
- encephalomyelitis
- neuropathy: motor neuronopathy, subacute sensory neuronopathy, sensorimotor neuropathy, and autonomic neuropathy
- MG, Eaton-Lambert syndrome
- myopathy: polymyositis, dermatomyositis, cachetic myopathy, neuromyotonia

Treatment: Tumour-ablation therapy is the most important. In MG and NMDAR encephalitis, where the associated tumours (thymoma and ovarian teratoma respectively) are completely resected, the prognosis is good. The prognosis is generally poor if the syndrome is associated to an inoperable tumour or incurable malignancy. Plasmapheresis, IVIG, corticosteroids, and immunosuppressants can confer transient relief or stabilization of symptoms.

Neurological complications of chemotherapy

The CNS is usually spared from neurotoxic effects of conventional chemotherapy agents because neuronal cells do not divide and because many agents cannot pass through the blood-brain-barrier unless it is disrupted. Drugs with different actions (e.g., hormonal and biological agents, monoclonal antibodies, small-molecule signal transduction inhibitors) are available. It is important to distinguish the adverse events of chemotherapy agents from those caused by the neoplasm.

Chemotherapy agent	Neurotoxic effects
Ifosfamide (alkylating agent)	• Encephalopathy, seizures • Cerebellar ataxia • Cranial neuropathies • Extrapyramidal dysfunction
Cisplatin (alkylating agent)	• Peripheral and cranial neuropathies • Paraesthesia in back and limbs with neck flexion • Encephalopathy, seizures, cortical blindness, loss of taste, SIADH
Methotrexate (dihydrofolate reductase inhibitor)	• Headaches, confusion, seizures • Chronic leukoencephalopathy with cognitive impairment months or years after exposure • Aseptic meningitis, myelopathy, acute encephalopathy (intrathecal administration)
5-Fluorouracil (fluorinated pyrimidine; thymidylate synthetase inhibitor)	• Acute cerebellar syndrome • Encephalopathy, seizures, optic neuropathy • Parkinsonian syndrome, focal dystonias
Cytosine arabinoside (pyrimidine analog; DNA polymerase inhibitor)	• Encephalopathy, seizures • Bulbar, pseudobulbar palsy • Aseptic meningitis, anosmia, extrapyramidal dysfunction
L-asparaginase (depletes L-asparagine)	• Sinus venous thrombosis, venous cerebral infarction

Neurological complications of radiotherapy

In radiotherapy, damage to adjacent structures may be unavoidable, e.g., temporal lobe or optic chiasmal damage from irradiation to NPC. Factors which determine the extent of damage include total dose, dose per fraction, duration of irradiation, and the individual's sensitivity to radiotherapy.

Complications can be:

- Acute (within days to several weeks of radiotherapy). Encephalopathy usually presents within 2 weeks, but can be within hours after cranial irradiation. It may present with nausea, vomiting, drowsiness, and headache. Corticosteroids are helpful.
- Early-delayed (1–6 months after radiotherapy). These include worsening of pre-existing neurological deficits, transient cognitive impairment, somnolence syndrome, brachial or lumbosacral plexopathy. The somnolence syndrome resolves in a few weeks.
- Late-delayed (years after radiotherapy). These include cerebral and spinal radionecrosis, leukoencephalopathy, brachial or lumbosacral plexopathy, cranial and motor neuropathy. Plexopathy tends to be progressive, and present with neuropathic pain and paraesthesia, wasting and weakness of affected muscles, and areflexia. MRI can help to distinguish between radiation-induced plexopathy and tumour recurrence. Corticosteroids and analgesics are used for symptomatic relief. Radionecrosis has become less common because of improved radiotherapy techniques. Predisposing factors of radionecrosis include pre-existing diabetes mellitus, associated chemotherapy, and old age. Corticosteroids and surgical excision of necrotic tissue may be indicated. Leukoencephalopathy is common in long-term cancer survivors, and is characterized by cognitive impairment associated with diffuse white matter abnormalities. In some patients, it may lead to progressive dementia, and the prognosis is generally poor.

NEUROTOXICITY

Effects of neurotoxins

- Constitutional: nausea, vomiting, fatigue, weight loss, insomnia
- CNS: altered mental state, dizziness, headache, personality change; stroke, seizure, ataxia, movement disorder, psychosis, and encephalopathy
- PNS: paraesthesia, visual and hearing loss, vertigo, autonomic dysfunction
- Neuromuscular junction and muscle: weakness, muscle cramps, myopathy

Environmental neurotoxins

Chemical elements

Lead

- Common source: paint, battery, petroleum, plastic industry
- Acute encephalopathy with headache, seizure or coma; more common in children
- Chronic poisoning results in asymmetric axonal polyneuropathy with predominant motor involvement.
- Diagnosed by raised blood or urine lead levels; gingival lead lines may be seen
- Specific treatment: chelation therapy using EDTA or dimercaprol or both

Arsenic

- Common source: insecticides, batteries
- Clinical signs: Mee's lines (transverse white lines at nail bed), palmar or plantar dermatitis or hyperkeratosis, garlic breath
- Acute encephalopathy may present with headache, vertigo, seizures, and coma.
- Chronic poisoning may result in sensorimotor neuropathy or optic neuropathy, muscle cramps and myalgia.

- Acute poisoning is diagnosed by abnormal increase in urine or blood arsenic levels. Hair and nail samples are useful for the diagnosis of chronic poisoning.
- Specific treatment: chelation therapy with dimercaprol

Mercury

- Common source: organic mercury from seafood contaminated by antifungal agents; inorganic mercury from paints, insecticides, and amalgam for dental fillings
- Clinical sign: gingival hypertrophy with bluish lines
- Acute poisoning: encephalopathy, psychosis, coma, myoclonus
- Chronic poisoning: encephalopathy, seizures, visual and hearing loss, neuropathy
- Painful neuropathy and autonomic dysfunction more common in children.
- Diagnosed by elevated mercury level in blood, urine or hair samples
- Specific treatment: chelation by dimercaprol or penicillamine. Ethylenediaminetetraacetic acid (EDTA) is contraindicated.

Manganese

- Source: metal welder, agricultural toxins, inhalation via environmental pollution or ingestion of polluted water
- Clinical features: parkinsonism, seizures, chronic encephalopathy
- Diagnosed by raised serum manganese level
- Specific treatment: EDTA chelation

Chemical compounds

Carbon monoxide

- Common source: charcoal combustion (suicide)
- Acute encephalopathy, seizure, coma, and delayed demyelination
- Chronic: headache, memory loss, tremor, ataxia, encephalopathy
- Clinical sign: anoxia without cyanosis, 'cherry-red' appearance
- Diagnosed by elevated carboxyhaemoglobin

- Severe cases require intubation and 100% oxygen. If available, hyperbaric oxygen, exchange transfusion, and induced hypothermia may be considered. Treat cerebral oedema and seizures, and provide supportive care.

Pesticides (e.g., organophosphates, cholinesterase inhibitors)

- Clinical features: nausea, vomiting, abdominal pain, bronchospasm, respiratory failure, paraesthesia, dysphagia, weakness
- Diagnosed by presence of organophosphates in gastric aspirate
- Specific antidotes: pralidoxine and atropine

Marine toxins

The clinical features following different forms of marine toxin poisoning are similar. Specific antidotes are not available and treatment is mainly supportive. A history of exposure and consistent clinical features are adequate for diagnosis.

Ciguatera poisoning

It is the most common form of marine poisoning which follows oral ingestion of ciguatoxins commonly found in reef and coral fish. Ciguatoxins are heat stable and activate voltage sensitive sodium channels. Symptoms are predominantly gastrointestinal (within 12–24 hours) or neurological (after 24 hours), including distal and perioral paraesthesia, myalgia, cold allodynia, and ataxia. Chronic poisoning may result in fatigue or anxiety-depression. There is no laboratory test to confirm exposure to cinguatoxins and the diagnosis is primarily clinical. NCV may be normal or show mild impairment.

Puffer fish (Tetrodotoxin) poisoning

It is the most common lethal marine poisoning, especially in Japan. Tetrodotoxin is stored mainly in the liver, ovary, and intestines. It is a water-soluble guanidine which binds to sodium channels and blocks impulse conduction. Symptoms of mild poisoning are similar to ciguatoxin. More severe cases develop distal, bulbar, and facial muscle weakness together with dizziness and ataxia. Life-threatening poisoning is characterized by respiratory failure, flaccid paralysis, coma, bradycardia, and hypotension. Analysis of uneaten fish or patient's urine for tetrodotoxin by high performance liquid chromatography can confirm the diagnosis. Treatment is supportive.

Shellfish

Paralytic shellfish poisoning is caused by saxitotoxin or gonyautoxins (derived from marine microalgae). The clinical picture is indistinguishable from tetrodotoxin poisoning. It occurs following ingestion of clams, oysters or mussels. The neuropathic form is caused by brevetoxins, and the encephalopathic form is caused by domic acid.

Substance abuse

- Alcohol
- Opiates: heroin, morphine, methadone, codeine, pethidine, propoxyphene
- Inhaled substances: gasoline, solvents, glue or paint containing hydrocarbons, e.g., n-hexane, toluene, nitrous oxide, trichloroethylene
- Sedatives and hypnotics: barbiturates, benzodiazepines
- CNS stimulants: cocaine (snow), amphetamines (speed), methylphenidate
- Hallucinogens: LSD, MDMA, phencyclidine (angel dust), ketamine (special K)
- Cannabis

Alcohol

Neurological complications include:
- Acute intoxication: euphoria, disinhibition, ataxia, stupor, respiratory depression

- Alcohol withdrawal: delirium tremens, seizures, tremors, hallucinations
- Alcoholic dementia
- Alcoholic cirrhosis with hepatic encephalopathy
- Wernicke's encephalopathy with or without Korsakoff syndrome
- Alcoholic cerebellar degeneration
- Central pontine myelinolysis
- Optic neuritis
- Polyneuropathy and myopathy
- Increased risk of stroke

Heroin

- It crosses the BBB rapidly and binds to specific opioid receptors (μ, δ, and κ) resulting in analgesia, miosis, respiratory suppression, and psychotropic effects.
- Acute effects: euphoria, intense relaxation, worry-free; apnoea, coma
- Complications are common: cellulitis, abscesses, osteomyelitis, endocarditis, septicaemia, meningitis, hepatitis B, C, and HIV; stroke, anoxic encephalopathy, rhabdomyolysis, nerve compression, and brachial plexopathy.
- Heroin overdose results in pinpoint pupils, coma, apnoea, hypotension, and hypothermia. Naloxone, a highly effective opioid antagonist, may reverse these effects.
- Opiate withdrawal syndrome consists of drug craving, irritability, sweating, lacrimation, rhinorrhoea, piloerection, abdominal cramps, and diarrhoea. These features may be suppressed by methadone or clonidine.

Solvents

- Includes benzene, ethylene glycol, n-hexane, acetone, and formaldehyde
- Exposure via recreational abuse or occupational contact, e.g., paint, gasoline or plastic industry
- Clinical features: encephalopathy, neuropathy, ataxia, movement disorder

- Specific treatment: activated charcoal for ingestion; dialysis to remove solvent; ethyl alcohol is a specific antidote of anti-freeze.

Benzodiazepines

- Acute effects: drowsiness, confusion, amnesia, euphoria, psychomotor slowing, coma, and rarely respiratory depression
- Flumazenil is a specific antidote which may be used to reverse coma.
- Chronic exposure very often leads to tolerance and dependence.
- Withdrawal symptoms include irritability, photophobia, phonophobia, sweating, tremor, tachycardia, headache, insomnia, delirium, hallucinations, and seizures. Reinstituting the benzodiazepine followed by slow withdrawal is the mainstay of treatment.

Cocaine

- Consumed by inhalation to bypass the first pass liver metabolism
- Enhances dopaminergic, serotoninergic, and noradrenergic transmission and has a local anaesthetic effect at mucous membrane
- Acute effects: increased energy, confidence, euphoria, and diminished sleep
- Toxicity includes cardiac arrhythmias, anxiety reaction, hypertension, cerebral haemorrhage, necrosis of nasal septum, foetal damage, and panic attack.

Amphetamines

- Currently used to treat narcolepsy and childhood attention deficit disorder
- Acute effects: tachycardia, arrhythmias, irritability, hallucinations, and psychosis
- Chronic exposure: strong psychological addiction, anxiety, depression

MDMA (3, 4-methylene dioxy-methamphetamine, Ecstasy)

- Causes serotonin release and blocks re-uptake and is structurally similar to amphetamine
- Acute effect: pleasurable agitation, decreased fatigue, feeling closeness to others; somatic effects include sweating, nausea, vomiting, and serotonin syndrome (dehydration, hyperthermia, and death).
- Chronic exposure: cognitive impairment, hepatotoxicity, severe hangover

Lysergic acid diethylamide (LSD)

- Structural resemblance to serotonin
- Acute ingestion results in euphoria, detachment, visual distortions, altered self-perception, dizziness, and tremor.
- Behavioural aberration, e.g., false belief of ability to fly resulting in fall from height
- Chronic exposure: flashbacks (vivid recollection of perceptual disturbance), persistent psychosis, depression

Cannabis (marijuana, dope, grass)

- Cannabis oil > resin > dried herbs in terms of potency
- Usually co-administered with tobacco
- Weak opiate-like and barbiturate-like effects
- Acute exposure results in mild euphoria, relaxation, altered time perception, increased appetite, mild tachycardia, and ataxia, progressing to paranoia, psychosis, and panic attacks in more severe cases.
- Chronic intoxication may cause anxiety, depression or relapse of schizophrenia.

_18_ Brain Tumours

Intracranial tumours may be benign or malignant, primary or secondary. Brain tumours in adults commonly occur above the tentorium cerebelli, in contrast to those in children that usually affect the cerebellum or brainstem. Since they may run a rapidly deteriorating course, brain tumours should be promptly diagnosed and appropriately treated. The classification of common intracranial tumours and their relative frequency are listed in Table 18.1.

Table 18.1   Classification and incidence

Tumour type	Age at presentation (y)	Site of predilection	Frequency (%)
Astrocytoma			40
– adult	40–60	Cerebral hemisphere	
– child	6–12	Optic nerve, cerebellum, hypothalamus, brainstem	
Oligodendroglioma	30–60	Cerebral hemisphere	3
Ependymoma	6–12	Lateral and IV ventricle	3
Medulloblastoma	5–15	IV ventricle, cerebellar vermis	3
Schwannoma	40–70	V and VIII cranial nerves	8
Meningioma	40–60	Dural surface, ventricle	18
Craniopharyngioma	5–60	Hypothalamus, III ventricle	2
Pituitary adenoma	Adult	Pituitary gland	10
Haemangioblastoma	5–60	Cerebellum	9
Metastatic*	Adult	Cerebral hemisphere	4
Lymphoma	Adult	Periventricular sites	< 0.5

*Cerebral metastasis commonly arises from primary carcinoma (of lung, breast, kidney, colon, choriocarcinoma)

Clinical features

Raised intracranial pressure (ICP)

- Mass effect (tumour, oedema, bleeding into tumour), shift of intracranial structures, obstructive hydrocephalus
- Diffuse headache with nausea, vomiting, visual blurring or papilloedema

Seizures

- Focal seizures, simple or complex, depending on the site of the tumour ± secondary generalization

Focal features of insidious onset and progressive course

- Depending on the site of the tumour
- Pressure effect, infiltration, or destruction
- False localizing signs: VI or III nerve palsy
- Frontal lobe dysfunction
  - intellectual decline or dementia
  - personality change, behavioural disturbance
  - expressive dysphasia (Broca) if lesion in the dominant hemisphere
  - motor deficits, e.g., hemiparesis, hyperreflexia, Babinski sign
  - Jacksonian seizures or partial motor seizures
  - urinary incontinence
  - release of primitive reflexes, e.g., grasping reflex, palmo-mental reflex, snouting response, rooting response, sucking response
  - anosmia or blindness from subfrontal lesions
- Temporal lobe dysfunction
  - memory impairment
  - receptive dysphasia (Wernicke) if lesion in the dominant hemisphere
  - complex partial seizures
  - homonymous upper quadrantanopia

- Parietal lobe dysfunction
  - cortical sensory loss (impaired two-point discrimination, astereognosis, sensory inattention)
  - dominant hemisphere signs (acalculia, agnosia, left-right disorientation, nominal dysphasia; Gerstmann's syndrome)
  - non-dominant hemisphere signs (ideomotor or dressing dyspraxia)
  - homonymous lower quadrantanopia
- Occipital lobe dysfunction
  - homonymous hemianopia
  - visual hallucination
  - visual agnosia or alexia
- Cerebellar and brainstem dysfunction
  - truncal ataxia in midline lesion
  - limb ataxia in hemispheric lesion
  - associated brainstem signs
  - obstructive hydrocephalus
  - cranial nerve deficits

Differential diagnosis

- Chronic subdural haematoma
- Infections, e.g., cerebral abscess, tuberculoma, cysticercosis, viral encephalitis
- Benign intracranial hypertension
- Cortical venous thrombosis

Investigations

- Plain radiography: skull X-ray (may show evidence of raised ICP or calcification); CXR (if cerebral metastasis is suspected)
- EEG: limited usefulness
- CT brain with contrast: useful for tumours with calcification, e.g., craniopharyngioma, meningioma (Figures 18.1a and 18.1b)
- MRI brain with gadolinium enhancement: better than CT in defining multiple small metastases and cranial nerve lesions, and in differentiating tumour from demyelination and abscess.

Magnetic resonance spectroscopy (MRS) may differentiate between tumour recurrence and radionecrosis.

- Digital subtraction angiography: for delineation of blood supply of tumours; as an adjunct to CT/MRI for exclusion of AVM. Pre-operative embolization of vascular tumours may be necessary.
- PET-CT is helpful in identifying the site of the primary tumour which has metastasized to the brain.

Management

1. Medical treatment is mainly supportive and consists of:
   - seizure control with AEDs
   - lowering ICP via reduction of oedema with IV or oral corticosteroids (dexamethasone or betamethasone) or IV mannitol
   - analgesics and antiemetics
2. Surgical treatment includes:
   - total tumour resection without producing neurological deficits especially for benign tumours
   - partial removal if critical areas (e.g., motor or language centre) are affected
   - stereotactic biopsy for tissue diagnosis
   - shunting to correct hydrocephalus, e.g., ventriculoperitoneal or temporary external drainage, fenestration by neuroendoscopy
3. Radiosurgery (gamma-knife, X-knife):
   - This is minimally invasive focal irradiation with stereotactic localization. Certain tumours (acoustic neuroma, metastasis) can be treated by this method when they are small. It is particularly suitable for tumours in surgically inaccessible sites or for patients who are unfit for major surgery.
4. Radiotherapy:
   - Radiosensitive tumours include medulloblastoma, pineal germinoma, ependymoma, and cerebellar cystic astrocytoma. High-grade malignant gliomas respond poorly to radiotherapy.

5. Chemotherapy:
   - Helpful in cerebral lymphoma or leukaemia and in certain primary intracranial tumours

SELECTED ENTITIES

Glioma

Gliomas (Figure 18.1c) are malignant intrinsic tumours from neuroglia of the brain. The cause is unknown. They spread via local extension without extracranial metastasis. Histological confirmation and grading of malignancy should be ascertained. Surgical excision may provide rapid relief of unpleasant symptoms. Adjuvant radiotherapy and chemotherapy increase survival.

Astrocytoma

- From astrocytes
- Grades I (slow growing) to IV (fast growing) according to degree of malignancy
- Cystic astrocytomas within the cerebellum in childhood; relatively benign

Oligodendroglioma

- From oligodendroglia
- Slow growing with calcification

Meningioma

- Arises from arachnoid membrane; mostly supratentorial in location (Figures 18.1a and 18.1b)
- May be static or slow growing. Mostly benign; may rarely become malignant
- Enhanced with contrast; calcification common

Neurofibroma

- Arises from Schwann cells of nerve sheath
- Usually located at the cerebellopontine angle

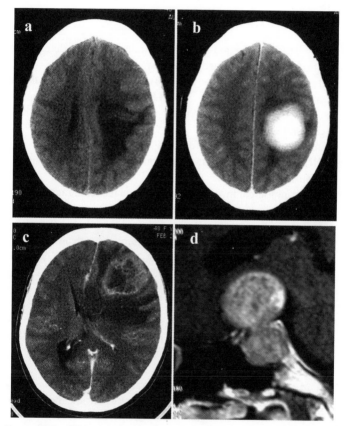

Figure 18.1 CT brain of a large supratentorial meningioma showing (a) a hypodense area with surrounding oedema and possibly some calcification on plain image and (b) intense enhancement with contrast; (c) CT brain with contrast showing a large frontal malignant glioma with ring-like enhancement, surrounding oedema, and mass effect; (d) gadolinium-enhanced sagittal T$_1$ weighted MRI pituitary and hypothalamus showing a large enhancing pituitary macroadenoma with suprasellar extension.

- VIII nerve most commonly involved, followed by V and IX nerves
- Multiple neurofibromas should raise suspicion of neurofibromatosis (Type I and II).

Pituitary tumour

- May be asymptomatic if small and non-secretory; detected on neuroimaging performed for other reasons
- May present with endocrine dysfunction or neurological features (including headache, visual blurring, or rarely apoplexy). A typical sign is bitemporal hemianopia or bilateral upper temporal quadrantanopia.
- Enlargement of pituitary fossa on lateral skull X-ray
- MRI (Figure 18.1d); high-resolution CT with coronal or sagittal reconstruction
- Endocrinological investigations: hormonal excess (acromegaly, Cushing's disease, hyperprolactinaemia); hormonal deficiency (pituitary dwarfism, hypothyroidism or hypoadrenalism)
- Common histological types: chromophobe adenomas (prolactinomas, non-functioning tumours), acidophil adenomas (secreting growth hormone), basophil adenomas (secreting ACTH)
- Treatment:
  - Surgical removal: trans-sphenoidal (small) or transfrontal (suprasellar extension or suspecting hypothalamic tumour); post-operative radiotherapy for incomplete removal
  - Radiosurgery: gamma-knife, X-knife
  - Medical treatment: dopamine agonists (for prolactinomas or growth hormone-producing tumour) to shrink the tumour; long-acting somatostatin analogues (octreotide) for acromegaly; inhibition of cortisol synthesis and release with 11-hydroxylase blocker (metyrapone or aminoglutethimide); replacement of hormone deficiency

Craniopharyngioma

- Cystic hypothalamic tumour from Rathke's pouch
- May be present at any age, but often in childhood
- Calcification is common
- Treatment: surgical excision; palliative stereotactic aspiration; palliative radiotherapy; palliative ventricular shunting

19 Neurorehabilitation

Neurorehabilitation is an integral part of the management of neurological disorders. Common disabling neurological conditions include stroke, Parkinson's disease, head and spinal cord trauma, epilepsy, brain and spinal cord tumours, and multiple sclerosis. Impairments include locomotion difficulty, hearing loss, visual impairment, cognitive impairment, behavioural disturbance, upper limb dysfunction, incontinence, and communication problems. Multiple domains are often affected.

Neurorehabilitation is a multidisciplinary effort to restore and enhance the highest possible functional level and quality of life for the patient and his family, whatever the cause or severity of the disability.

Rehabilitation team

1. Physicians/neurologists
    To assess functional disability and formulate a rehabilitation programme; to lead the team and to co-ordinate different members in the provision of seamless patient care.

2. Nurses
    To provide nursing care, e.g., bowel and bladder management, skin care; may assist in co-ordinating the rehabilitation team; to ensure that skills learned from therapists are passed to the nursing unit.

3. Physiotherapists
    To assess physical disability; to strengthen muscles, improve mobility, and prevent or reduce contractures. Physical modalities such as short-wave, ultrasound, ice, hot pad, and

electrotherapy may be used for pain relief. EMG biofeedback, weight-supported treadmill training, or functional electrical stimulation may also be used to augment training effect.

4. Occupational therapists

   To assess and provide training in activities of daily living (ADL). The Barthel index (Table 19.1) is commonly used. Interventions include the provision of aids (e.g., simple hand orthosis, splints), tools for daily living, wheelchair prescription, advice on alteration of environment at home and at work, vocational evaluation, home assessment, perceptual assessment, and cognitive rehabilitation.

5. Speech therapists

   To assess patient's level of communication; to teach non-verbal communication skills and provide communication aids; to deal with problems of swallowing.

6. Clinical psychologists

   To administer neuropsychometric evaluation (for intellect, memory, mood, comprehension, and expression); to help set realistic goals and teach coping strategies and behavioural modification; to provide counselling to patients and family members.

7. Medical social workers

   To liaise with relatives and provide counselling; to advise on legal guardianship; to obtain social welfare for patients; to co-ordinate discharge planning and provide continuity of contact in the community after discharge.

8. Vocational counsellors

   To minimize the delay in starting work following successful rehabilitation.

9. Voluntary organizations, e.g., self-help groups

   To provide financial support or equipment, organize educational seminars, and encourage fellowship among patients and carers.

10. Personnel in related specialties, e.g., ophthalmologists, audiologists, ENT surgeons, urologists, orthotists, orthopaedic surgeons.

Table 19.1   Barthel (ADL) index

Bowels	Transfer
0 = Incontinent	0 = Unable
1 = Occasional accident	1 = Major help (1–2 people, physical)
2 = Continent	2 = Minor help (verbal or physical)
	3 = Independent
Bladder	
0 = Incontinent or catheterized	**Mobility**
1 = Occasional accident	0 = Immobile
2 = Continent	1 = Independent in wheelchair
	2 = Walks with help of 1 person
Dressing	3 = Independent walking
0 = Dependent	
1 = Needs help, but can do half unaided	**Grooming**
2 = Independent	0 = Needs help
	1 = Independent
Toilet use	
0 = Dependent	**Stairs**
1 = Needs some help	0 = Unable
2 = Independent	1 = Needs help
	2 = Independent up and down
Feeding	
0 = Unable	**Bathing**
1 = Needs help, e.g., spreading butter	0 = Dependent
2 = Independent	1 = Independent

Total Score _____

20	Full physical independence
16–19	Mildly disabled
10–15	Moderately disabled
5–9	Severely disabled
0–4	Very severely disabled

Paradigms in neurorehabilitation

CNS plasticity

Some degree of neurological recovery is often observed after neural injury. Possible mechanisms include:
• Synaptic reorganization
• Unmasking of latent neural pathways
• Sprouting of nerve terminals
• Alteration of receptors and neurotransmitters

Before instituting rehabilitation, ascertain:

1. Pathology
2. Impairment
3. Disability
4. Handicap

A typical example is a patient who had cerebral infarction due to occlusion of the left MCA (the pathology), causing right hemiparesis and dysphasia (the impairments). The latter results in difficulty in mobility and communication (the disability), and problems with social adjustment, e.g., unemployment, dependent ADL, and loss of usual social activities (the handicap).

Impairments may improve within a period of time (e.g., 1–2 years for head injury), but thereafter become permanent. No treatment can reverse impairments. However, rehabilitation can help improve disability and handicap, and hence quality of life. Rehabilitation may benefit even serious and fatal conditions such as MND.

Goals

1. Prevention of complications
2. Promotion of neurological recovery
3. To teach adaptive skills
4. Facilitation of environmental interaction

The goals should be realistic and achievable and the programme tailored to this end for the patient. There is no point in an overdose of rehabilitation in the hope of achieving the unachievable.

Specific impairments that may benefit from rehabilitation

1. Cognitive impairment
   - Training to follow instructions; matching and selecting tasks; sorting and sequencing exercises
   - Enhancing memory performance by interactive visual imagery, cueing, writing diaries and notes

2. Dysphasia
   - Rote learning and selective stimulation
   - Use of cues; operant conditioning; rhythm therapy
   - Verbal communication aids/systems based on printed materials or hand gestures

3. Dysphagia
   - Not uncommon in neurologically impaired patients
   - Avoid aspiration and pneumonia particularly in those with bulbar dysfunction; aspiration may be silent.
   - Special investigations, e.g., videofluoroscopic swallowing study, fibreoptic endoscopic evaluation of swallowing
   - Nasogastric tube feeding as a temporary measure; percutaneous gastrostomy as a long-term measure
   - Modified diet prescription to enable some patients to resume oral feeding

4. Dysarthria
   - Increase patient's awareness of mild deficits to allow for autocompensation
   - Exercise to improve weak orofacial muscles
   - Communication aids may be used in patients with severe dysarthria

5. Hearing impairment
   - Hearing aids: distortion may be troublesome.
   - Amplification devices fitted to phone, radio or TV; personal alarm devices

6. Spasticity
   - Removal of nociceptive stimuli, e.g., faecal impaction, bedsore, and cystitis; proprioceptive facilitation
   - Physical therapy including prolonged stretching of spastic muscles and active limb exercises
   - Useful drugs including diazepam, baclofen, and dantrolene
   - More refractory and severe cases may require nerve block, botulinum toxin injection, and intrathecal baclofen administered via a lumbar catheter.
   - Surgical division of soft tissues may be indicated for disabling contractures.

7. Motor weakness (hemiplegia, tetraplegia or paraplegia)
   - Quantitative grading of muscle power by the Medical Research Council (MRC) system (Table 19.2)
   - Concomitant effect of spasticity should be considered.
   - Passive and active physiotherapy in different phases of rehabilitation
   - Rigid orthosis and crutches for patients with conus lesion
   - Reciprocating gait orthosis for higher lesion
   - Functional electrical stimulation
   - Wheelchairs: indoor *vs* outdoor use ± accessories

Table 19.2   Medical Research Council (MRC) scale

Grade	Description
0	No contraction
1	Flicker of contraction
2	Active movement when gravity eliminated
3	Active movement against gravity
4−	Active movement against gravity with slight resistance
4	Active movement against gravity with moderate resistance
4+	Active movement against gravity with strong resistance
5	Normal power

8. Neuropathic bladder
   - Complications: recurrent urinary tract infection, vesico-ureteric reflux, ureteric obstruction ± renal failure, urinary calculi, and autonomic dysfunction (autonomic dysreflexia)
   - Bladder hyperactivity ± secondary outlet obstruction: anticholinergics to suppress detrusor activity, bladder cystoplasty
   - Bladder hypoactivity: cholinergics (e.g., bethanecol), prostaglandins
   - Hyperactive urethra: spasmolytics, α-blockers, sphincterotomy
   - Sphincter incompetence: α-agonists, implantable artificial sphincters
   - Intermittent or permanent catheterization
   - Regular timing for toiletting and fluid intake advice
   - Other measures for urinary incontinence: pants and absorbent pads, occlusive devices for male patients, drainage appliances (e.g., condom sheath)

9. Neurogenic bowel
   - Results in constipation and/or incontinence
   - Drug treatment for constipation: bulking agents, stool softeners, stimulants, osmotics or rectal suppositories
   - Bowel training programme: regular toilet regime to capitalize on gastrocolic reflex; digital stimulation
   - Manual evacuation
   - Anal sphincter repair; dynamic graciloplasty; permanent colostomy
   - Artificial bowel sphincter
   - Pads and pants; anal plug for faecal incontinence

20 Common Medicolegal Issues in Neurology

In certain neurological conditions, often rapidly evolving or trauma-related, doctors (in particular those in the emergency room, surgical or medical ward, as well as family physicians) may be involved in providing factual evidence or as subjects of complaints or medical negligence actions. The purpose of this chapter is to enhance awareness rather than to provide comprehensive coverage.

In the management of neurological or neurosurgical disorders, it is essential to ensure detailed history taking, thorough examination, quality care, and contemporaneous documentation (of relevant positive and negative findings, diagnosis, management, and communication with patients and relatives).

Head injury

Head injury is a major cause of death and morbidity. In most cases, two forms of brain damage occur: primary and secondary. The injury (blunt, penetrating or rapid deceleration) produces primary damage to the brain. Following the primary injury, the brain is vulnerable to secondary damage (oedema, hypoxia, ischaemia, haemorrhage), which may occur within minutes. Systemic injuries also contribute to secondary damage of the brain. In severe head injury, respiratory compromise (due to chest injuries, airway obstruction, and/or depressant drugs) is common, resulting in hypoxia and hypercapnia. Brain hypoxia may also result from blood loss and hypotension. Treatment must be directed at preventing or reducing the effects of these secondary complications.

Sequelae in the acute stage

Soft-tissue and skull injuries

In the face and scalp, injuries range from bruising to lacerations, and the wound may be contaminated.

Linear skull fracture rarely requires specific treatment. Compound depressed fracture tends to be associated with localized brain damage. In such cases, the dura may be torn with the attendant risk of infection (e.g., abscess or meningitis), and the brain may be lacerated. Osteitis may follow skull fracture (depressed or non-depressed), the usual organism being staphylococcus. Penetrating skull injuries often require surgery.

Dural tears should be suspected if CSF leaks from the fracture site, nose or ears, in the presence of meningitis, or if intracranial air is shown on X-ray or CT.

Intracranial haematoma (Figure 20.1)

- Epidural haematoma commonly due to tear of the middle meningeal artery
- Subdural haematoma may be acute, subacute or chronic.
- Intracerebral haematomas are usually multifocal and situated in the frontal and temporal lobes. Acute cerebral contusion may evolve into a haematoma, and delayed cerebral haemorrhage is a well-recognized feature in head injury.

The clinical effects of the haematoma may be immediate but may also be delayed for several hours or even days. It usually presents as deterioration in consciousness. Urgent evacuation is often required for acute intracranial haematoma, especially the epidural variety.

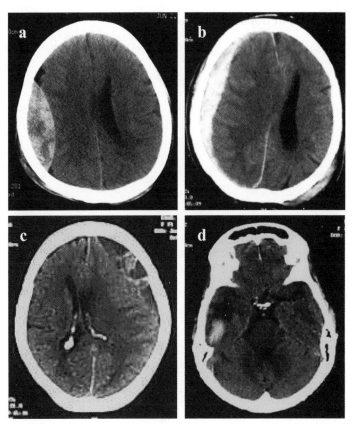

Figure 20.1   CT brain showing (a) an acute right epidural haematoma,
(b) an acute right subdural haematoma, and (c) a chronic left subdural
haematoma. Note compression of the ipsilateral cerebral hemisphere
and lateral ventricle; midline shift also present in (b) and (c). (d) CT
brain showing right temporal lobe contusion with cerebral oedema
surrounding the traumatic intracerebral haematoma.

Primary parenchymal damage

Cerebral contusion is focal or multifocal, commonly situated at the frontal and temporal poles.

Diffuse axonal injury is often associated with severe impairment of consciousness. The probable mechanism is shearing injury of the white matter. Multiple petechial haemorrhages are better visualized on MRI than CT.

The cranial nerves, especially I, II, IV, and VI, may be damaged.

Cerebral oedema

Two types of cerebral oedema may occur. Vasogenic oedema is due to an increase in extracellular fluid as a result of increased permeability of cerebral capillaries. It tends to be associated with a focal lesion, e.g., haematoma. Cytotoxic oedema results from an increase in intracellular fluid and is related to diffuse brain hypoxia.

Vascular damage

Cerebral blood vessels may be damaged, resulting in traumatic aneurysm (with or without rupture), dissection (with or without arterial occlusion), or carotico-cavernous fistula.

Systemic complications

Stress gastric ulcers and aspiration pneumonia may develop after severe head injury. Inappropriate central sympathetic discharges may result in labile blood pressure and cardiac arrhythmia.

Long-term sequelae

Global and focal deficits

As a result of damage to the brain parenchyma and cranial nerves, global dysfunction (e.g., persistent vegetative state, cognitive, emotional, and behavioural disturbances), and focal deficits (e.g., dysphasia, deafness, anosmia, blindness, diplopia, hemiparesis, and movement disorders) may occur. However, it is imperative that reversible causes (e.g., chronic hydrocephalus, chronic subdural haematoma) should be excluded.

Post-concussion syndrome

Concussion refers to mild diffuse cerebral injury with altered consciousness. The post-concussion syndrome usually occurs during the recovery period following mild head injuries. The patient may have headache, dizziness, poor concentration, subjective cognitive and memory deficits, and may be irritable, anxious or depressed. The headache is usually described as heaviness or a band around the head, but intracranial complications should be excluded if it is severe or associated with focal neurological deficits. The symptoms usually resolve within a year in the majority of patients but may become chronic in a minority.

Post-traumatic epilepsy

Seizures may develop after head injury as early (within the first 7 days) or late post-traumatic epilepsy. Patients with severe head injury, in particular those with loss of consciousness for over 24 hours, intracranial haematoma, and cerebral contusion, are at greater risk of developing seizures.

History and examination

It is essential to obtain a detailed history, including the nature and timing of the injury, the sequence of events, and associated symptoms. A careful baseline documentation of all physical injuries and clinical signs is vital. The conscious level should be recorded using the GCS. Impaired consciousness in a drunken person should not be solely attributed to alcohol intoxication. In patients with suspected complications of head injury, regular neurological observation is mandatory. Associated neck, orthopaedic, intra-thoracic, and abdominal injuries are common particularly in falls from height and in motor vehicle accidents.

Post-traumatic amnesia (PTA) or anterograde amnesia may be defined as an absence of continuous memory or inability to retain new information following head injury. The duration of loss of consciousness and PTA correlate with the severity of head injury and should be accurately documented. Retrograde amnesia refers to loss of memory for events immediately before the head injury and is usually of short duration.

Investigations

In mild head injury, skull X-ray can be performed to look for fractures. However, a normal skull X-ray does not obviate the need for clinical observation especially in patients with suspected complications. In moderate or severe head injury, CT is the main investigation. Not only can it detect most intracranial traumatic lesions, but skull fractures are also visualized in bone window images. In some cases, MRI is better than CT in detecting brain oedema, cerebral herniation or brainstem compression. Occasionally, angiography may be performed if intracranial and extracranial vascular injuries are suspected. Injuries of the neck and other internal organs, if any, should also be assessed and investigated as appropriate.

Principles of management

It is not possible to admit every patient with head injury. However, if a full initial assessment is not possible (e.g., in young children, those with alcohol or drug abuse), or if complications are suspected, the patient should be admitted for observation. The likelihood of complication is increased if any of the following features is present: altered consciousness for more than a brief period, PTA, seizures, focal neurological deficit, and skull fracture. Patients with head injury are generally taken care of by neurosurgeons.

Specific treatments include:

- Monitoring and control of ICP
- Evacuation of intracranial haematoma

– Maintenance of adequate cerebral perfusion
– Prevention and treatment of seizures

Supportive and general treatments include:

– Maintenance of airway and adequate ventilation
– Haemodynamic support
– Treatment for systemic injuries
– Prevention of pressure sores and contractures

Stroke

Subarachnoid haemorrhage

In its classical presentation, SAH is not difficult to diagnose (see Chapter 6). Cases which may be missed are those with a sentinel bleed due to leakage from an aneurysm. The headache may be severe at onset, but often resolves at the time of consultation. The patient is asymptomatic and without neck rigidity. CT brain may not show subarachnoid blood. The clinical clue in such cases is the sudden, severe, explosive or unaccustomed headache. With such history, even though CT is negative, LP should be considered. MRA aids the diagnosis by showing the aneurysm. Timely diagnosis is of particular importance as prompt surgical intervention will pre-empt a serious and potentially fatal recurrent bleed.

Dissection of cerebral arteries (see Chapter 6)

CNS infections (see Chapter 13)

The majority of pyogenic meningitis presents in the classical way. The difficulty is not with the diagnosis, but rather with timely treatment. In any suspected case of pyogenic meningitis, empirical antibiotics in meningitic dosage should be given after blood culture. No time should be wasted in arranging LP or awaiting results of CSF analysis. However, in cases of meningococcal meningitis, even such prompt treatment may not avert mortality or serious morbidity.

Chronic meningitis (tuberculous, fungal, neoplastic) is more difficult to diagnose, given the insidious onset and non-specific symptoms. However, in patients with an immunocompromised state or underlying malignancy, chronic meningitis should be considered in the presence of recent onset of headache, impaired consciousness or cranial nerve palsy. The typical CSF findings would assist the diagnosis.

Viral encephalitis may present with psychiatric features, resulting in delayed or wrong diagnosis. As a rule, functional disorders should not be diagnosed unless organic conditions have been carefully excluded. EEG is helpful in such cases.

Brain death (see Chapter 12)

Vegetative state and minimally conscious state (see Chapter 12)

Spinal cord trauma

- Commonly due to motor vehicle or industrial accidents, falls, sporting injuries, or violence
- Mechanisms: direct cord contusion; secondary to spine injury (fracture dislocation, subluxation). Patients with pre-existing narrow spinal canal and/or spondylosis are more prone to develop spinal cord deficits upon trauma.
- Immediate onset of symptoms, with presentation depending on the magnitude and site of impact
- In the first-aid management of accident victims, consider the possibility of neck injury and stabilize the cervical spine with a collar.
- The site of cord trauma determines the deficits. A high cervical cord lesion may bring about respiratory distress in addition to tetraparesis. A low cervical cord lesion would bring about mixed UMN and LMN weakness of the upper limbs and UMN

weakness of the lower limbs, as well as a level below which sensations are impaired or lost. A thoracic cord trauma would give rise to spastic paraparesis and a sensory level. A conus/cauda equina lesion, commonly due to fracture dislocation of the lower thoracic and upper lumbar vertebrae, would bring about corresponding features (see Figure 14.1).

- Investigations include X-ray, MRI, and CT of the relevant region of the spine. Care must be taken not to aggravate any instability or malalignment of the cervical spine.
- Urgent administration of IV high dose steroids may ameliorate cord damage. Surgery on the spine is indicated if there is instability or malalignment, or spinal cord compression due to protruded disc or bone fragments.
- Complications in the acute stage include respiratory insufficiency, pneumonia, urinary tract infection, deep vein thrombosis, and bedsores; these should be actively prevented or treated.
- Long-term complications include neurogenic bladder, urinary infection, renal calculi, renal failure, pressure sores, autonomic dysreflexia, heterotopic ossification, contractures, and pulmonary problems. Post-traumatic syringomyelia should be suspected if there is neurological deterioration after a stable period. MRI is the investigation of choice. Effective surgical treatment is available.

Whiplash injury

- This term refers to a collection of symptoms following injury to the neck, usually hyperextension-flexion, often the result of motor accident. Late whiplash syndrome (LWS) occurs in a small percentage of victims of whiplash injury and refers to a state in which the symptoms persist for more than 6 months after the accident.
- The symptoms include neck pain and stiffness, headache, dizziness, visual disturbance, pain, and paraesthesia in the upper limbs, subjective cognitive deficits, irritability, anxiety, and depression.

- Little or no objective evidence of damage to the nervous system (i.e., brain, spinal cord, spinal roots) can be elicited. The symptoms are due to injuries to the soft tissues and cervical spine.
- The pathological nature of the cognitive and psychiatric symptoms in LWS is still debated. The different views include psychoneurosis, psychosocial influences, pain-induced behaviour, and malingering.
- Whiplash injury may lead to premature development of cervical spondylosis, but there is no evidence that CSM or CSR are more common in subjects with whiplash injury than those without.
- Explanation of the nature of the symptoms, repeated reassurance of the absence of neurological damage, muscle relaxants, analgesics, and physiotherapy are helpful.

Cauda equina compression by lumbar prolapsed intervertebral disc (see Chapter 14)

Sciatic nerve injury

This is a common medical negligence claim. The sciatic nerve is injured when an IM injection is administered at the buttock, either through direct needle puncture or the injection of an irritant drug, e.g., NSAID, steroids, benzodiazepines.

The patient would experience pain and weakness in the sciatic nerve innervated dermatomes and muscles during or immediately after the injection. Later on, the typical clinical features consist of wasting and weakness of the leg and foot muscles, foot drop, and sensory disturbance over the lateral aspect of the leg and dorsum of foot. Disabling neuralgia may occur in some cases. The injected drug, if irritant, may also cause necrosis or atrophy of soft tissues at and around the injection site. Recovery is partial in most cases and may take months. In general, specific treatment is not available. Physiotherapy and occupational therapy are adjunctive measures.

The standard teaching for IM injection at the buttock is to administer the injection at the upper outer quadrant of the buttock with the patient in a lying position. Even so, the sciatic nerve may occasionally be injured because of anatomical variations. Injection with the patient in a sitting position increases the chances of sciatic nerve injury because of distorted anatomical landmarks. Thus, the lateral thigh has been recommended as the least unsafe IM injection site because there is no major nerve or blood vessel traversing that area. The need for IM administration of drugs should also be carefully evaluated.

Further Reading

Brazis, P. W., Masdeu, J. C., and Biller, J. *Localization in Clinical Neurology*. 6th ed. Philadelphia, PA: Wolters Kluwer, 2011.

Daroff, R. B., Fenichel, G. M., Jankovic J., and Maziotta, J. *Bradley's Neurology in Clinical Practice*. 6th ed. Philadelphia, PA: Elsevier, 2012.

Donaghy, M. (ed.). *Brain's Diseases of the Nervous System*. 12th ed. Oxford: Oxford University Press, 2009.

Dyck, P. J., and Thomas, P. K. *Peripheral Neuropathy*. 4th ed. Philadelphia, PA: Elsevier Saunders, 2005.

Engel, A., and Franzini-Armstrong, C. *Myology*. 3rd ed. New York: McGraw-Hill, 2004.

Glick, T. H. *Neurologic Skills: Examination and Diagnosis*. Boston, MA: Blackwell Scientific Publications, 1993.

Grotta, J. C., Albers, G. W., Broderick, J., et al. (eds.). *Stroke: Pathophysiology, Diagnosis and Management*. 6th ed. Philadelphia, PA: Elsevier, 2016.

Ropper, A. H., Gress. D. R., Diringer, M. N., et al. *Neurological and Neurosurgical Intensive Care*. 5th ed. Philadelphia, PA: Lippincott Williams & Wilkins, 2014.

Ropper, A. H., Samuels, M. A., and Klein, J. P. *Adams and Victor's Principles of Neurology*. 10th ed. New York: McGraw-Hill Education Medical, 2014.

Wyllie E., Cascino, G. D., Gidal, B. E., and Goodkin, H. P. (eds.). *Wyllie's Treatment of Epilepsy: Principles and Practice*. 5th ed. Philadelphia, PA: Lippincott Williams & Wilkins, 2011.

Index

Note: f = figure; t = table